Matters of Life and Death

PUBLIC HEALTH ISSUES IN CANADA

André Picard

D0043224

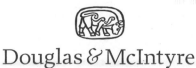

Douglas & McIntyre

1 2 3 4 5 — 21 20 19 18 17

DOUGLAS AND MCINTYRE (2013) LTD.
P.O. Box 219, Madeira Park, BC, V0N 2H0
www.douglas-mcintyre.com

Edited by Arlene Prunkl
Indexed by Emma Skagen
Cover design by Anna Comfort O'Keeffe
Text design by Shed Simas / Onça Design
Printed and bound in Canada

Canada Council   Conseil des arts
for the Arts   du Canada

BRITISH COLUMBIA
ARTS COUNCIL
An agency of the Province of British Columbia

Douglas and McIntyre (2013) Ltd. acknowledges the support of the Canada Council for the Arts, which last year invested $153 million to bring the arts to Canadians throughout the country. We also gratefully acknowledge financial support from the Government of Canada through the Canada Book Fund and from the Province of British Columbia through the BC Arts Council and the Book Publishing Tax Credit.

LIBRARY AND ARCHIVES CANADA CATALOGUING IN PUBLICATION

Picard, André, 1960-, author
        Matters of life and death : public health issues in Canada / André Picard.

Includes index.
Issued in print and electronic formats.
ISBN 978-1-77162-154-0 (softcover).--ISBN 978-1-77162-155-7 (HTML)

        1. Public health--Canada. 2. Medical policy--Canada. I. Title.

RA395.C3P53 2017   362.10971   C2017-900900-1
                                                     C2017-900901-X

Table of Contents

Introduction

I've had the privilege of being a reporter and columnist at *The Globe and Mail* for more than thirty years. Although I did a stint on general assignment (as all rookies must) and was preoccupied with Quebec politics during the tumultuous pre-referendum era, most of my time has been spent writing about health issues.

I don't have a background in medicine or health. I studied business administration, with a specialty in accounting, and then journalism. I also worked for several years in the student press. I stumbled into the health field quite by accident. When I began working at the *Globe* as a summer intern in 1987, AIDS was just beginning to become a mainstream news story. It was a time when many people—most of them gay men—were dying in large numbers, when treatments were virtually non-existent and when discrimination was rampant. It was also a time of much anger and many protests. Militant groups like ACT-UP (AIDS Coalition to Unleash Power) not only challenged scientists and politicians to do more in response to the out-of-control epidemic, but they forced media to rethink how they write about health care. At the time, medical reporting was very deferent: scientists published research in august journals, and those findings were reported, mostly uncritically. The notion that patients would have an opinion, let alone a legitimate one, was largely unthinkable. AIDS activists demanded to be heard, and that forever changed health-care delivery—and health journalism.

Of the thousands of stories I've written over the years, a handful have left an indelible mark on me. One of them was the story of a man admitted to St. Michael's Hospital in Toronto for treatment of a bacterial infection. He had not been tested for AIDS, and his condition was in no way related to a sexually transmitted disease. Yet because he was openly gay, the hospital affixed a sign above his bed—printed in bold type on bright pink cardboard, no less—reading: "Warning: risk of blood and body fluid contamination." When I visited him, I reached out to shake his hand, and he burst into tears. That was because many physicians and nurses had refused to touch him; his meals were left at the door because staff would not enter the room. After that story ran, St. Mike's apologized publicly and changed its policy so such discriminatory signs were banned. It went on to become one of the leading centres in the country, if not the world, for treating people with HIV-AIDS.

That encounter taught me two invaluable lessons. First, good health care requires a lot more than medicine and technology; it's about treating people with dignity and respect, and without judgment. Second, if journalism is going to be useful and impactful, it needs to look beyond the theoretical findings of scientists and the technical abilities of physicians and focus on the patient experience in the real world. Put another way, health policy and health politics matter as much as medicine. And what distinguishes my writing—stories and columns alike—from that of other health journalists is that I focus on policy rather than medicine.

The most impactful journalism I have done in my career is coverage of the tainted-blood scandal. This came about, as many good stories do, from asking a simple question. In the 1980s, the crude shorthand we used to remember the groups at high risk for HIV-AIDS was the "4H Club"—homosexuals, Haitians, heroin users and hemophiliacs. Each of those groups was getting extensive coverage, save one—hemophiliacs. A little digging revealed that people with clotting disorders, who routinely injected blood products to control their symptoms, were at extremely high risk. So too were people who underwent surgery. The numbers were mind-boggling: testing showed that almost half of all hemophiliacs had contracted the AIDS virus along with thousands of surgery patients. But very little was written about the risks of transfusion of blood and blood products, and what was written turned out to be based largely on egregious lies. The Canadian Red Cross stated publicly and repeatedly that the risk of contracting HIV from blood was "less than one in a million," and Health Canada, responsible for regulating the safety of drugs, went along unquestioningly. Yet before testing was implemented, after delays designed to use up stocks to save money, the risk was as high as 1 in 266. Tainted blood turned out to be the worst public-health disaster in Canadian history—and one of the worst in the world. More than twenty-four hundred hemophiliacs and transfusion recipients were infected with HIV-AIDS, and another twenty thousand or so contracted hepatitis C from blood and blood products. The revelations in *The Globe and Mail* led to a public inquiry, headed by Mr. Justice Horace Krever, and compensation of almost $5 billion to the victims and their families.

Yet the real tragedy of tainted blood is that the carnage was in large part preventable. Sadly, despite the enormity of the scandal, it was covered only retrospectively; it went virtually unnoticed for almost a decade after the first victims started dying. In 1994, I was invited to address a conference of the Canadian Association of Journalists on the topic, "Could the media have done a better job covering the tainted-blood tragedy?" I said this: "We journalists are guilty of the same 'crime' as the main players in the blood system … a failure to inform the public. Like them, we have excuses, but collectively our mistakes have cost hundreds, maybe thousands, of people their lives. There can be no excuse for that. We cannot be forgiven. But we can learn from our failures by never repeating them again."

Over the years, I have covered many issues, from AIDS through to Zika. This book is a selection of those columns, slightly updated to ensure they are current, though when I first discussed this idea with the publisher, I said, only half-jokingly, "The good news is that in Canadian health care, nothing ever changes, so even old columns are still current." Of course, the bad news is that in Canadian health care, nothing ever changes.

But to be fair, that isn't really true. Health care is immeasurably better today than when I started writing about it three decades ago. But our expectations are much higher. And the system is not adapting nearly quickly enough to profound changes in demographics, technology and medicine. It's a constant game of catch-up where we fall a little bit further behind every day. It's like that in journalism, too, an industry and a profession that has undergone cataclysmic change in recent years. Today, the good health reporting is better than it's ever been, but the bad health reporting is worse than it's ever been. If nothing else, at least the good health journalists have become more introspective and self-critical.

A few years back, Gary Schwitzer, a former medical correspondent at CNN and the founder of *Health News Review*, a health-news watchdog newsletter, penned a list of ten troublesome trends in health news. Most people today get their health information from the media and from television in particular. This places a heavy responsibility on journalists. But in Schwitzer's estimation, health reporting has many shortcomings, which he summarized like this:

1) *Too brief to matter.* The brevity of stories—they rarely exceed one minute on TV or five hundred words in print—means they lack context and significant details.
2) *No full-time health journalists.* Networks such as the CBC and CTV and newspapers such as *The Globe and Mail* have full-time beat reporters, but they are the exceptions. Most media outlets operate on the wrong-headed assumption that any reporter can jump effortlessly from covering city hall to the intricacies of cyclo-oxygenase-2 inhibitors.
3) *No data to back up sensational claims.* Far too many unproven—and at times frankly ridiculous—claims are aired or printed without even the most cursory examination of data.

4) *Hyperbole.* Each day reports of miracle drugs and treatments appear that in fact are, at best, incremental improvements.
5) *Commercialism.* At times, health "news" is thinly veiled promotional material.
6) *Single sources.* Health stories with just a single source are commonplace. They lack balance.
7) *Baseless predictions from basic science.* Far too many studies conducted in test tubes or on mice are touted as potential treatments in people. If only it were so simple.
8) *FDA approval treated as an accomplished fact.* Consumers are often left with the impression that experimental treatments and drugs in early phases of research will be on the market imminently, as if testing and regulatory approval are mere formalities.
9) *Little coverage of health policy.* Trivialities like cosmetic medicine (Botox and the like) get more coverage than critical issues like access to care and defining what is in the medicare "basket of services."
10) *No time for enterprise.* Much health reporting is little more than regurgitation of news releases, medical journal studies and press conferences. There is little investment in in-depth or investigative journalism.

Mr. Schwitzer's list is a good one, but it is incomplete. Here are ten more troublesome trends:

1) *Story selection.* Cute trumps meaningful. Quirky or pathos-laden stories, such as the separation of conjoined twins, tend to get more extensive coverage than those with broad policy implications, such as research questioning the value of breast cancer screening.
2) *Black and white.* Health stories tend to be black or white. Vioxx bad; Aspirin good. Trans fats bad; omega-3s good. But in science and health research a lot of greys exist; there are rarely absolutes.

3) *Jingoism.* The media give disproportionate attention to homegrown research, regardless of the importance or relevance of findings.

4) *Short-sightedness.* There is virtually no coverage of the greatest threats to health on the planet: poverty, disenfranchisement and lack of access to clean water, adequate nutrition and basic sanitation.

5) *Too little training.* Much research published in medical journals is of dizzying complexity and its jargon is quasi-impenetrable. Journalists need to understand statistics and technical language to decipher it, but media outlets are reluctant to invest in training.

6) *Obsession with technology.* A widespread assumption exists in health stories that newer is better, and that the solution to many problems is found in newer drugs and fancier equipment. Again, the reality is that addressing basic determinants of health—income, housing and the like—carries far more impact.

7) *Is it really a cure?* The word *cure* is bandied about irresponsibly. We have many ways of treating and managing disease, but virtually no cures. And "curing" a rat of cancer is a far cry from curing it in a human.

8) *A sense of proportion.* SARS killed forty-four people in Canada. Influenza and pneumonia kill close to five thousand annually. Health issues that affect the economy and the lives of well-to-do Westerners are blown out of proportion compared with issues that affect broad swaths of the population.

9) *Lack of skepticism.* One of the most important traits for journalists is a well-honed sense of doubt—about everything. When skepticism makes way for cheerleading, the result is poor health reporting.

10) *Kowtowing.* A lot of uncritical reporting occurs of the views of those in positions of power—physicians, professors, medical associations and pharmaceutical company executives—without questioning their self-interest. This pandering does a great disservice to health consumers.

Good health reporting should provide a straightforward, comprehensible summary of health issues. It has to be more than regurgitation. It needs to be balanced and provide context to information-hungry consumers. It has to take complex issues and make them digestible and relevant. Good health reporting should rarely be sensational, but always be skeptical. We can't forget that the issues we write about are important to patients, their families, policy-makers, politicians, clinicians and scientists. Often, seemingly banal issues turn out to be matters of life and death.

CHAPTER 1

Medicare

Dragging medicare into the
twenty-first century

Nothing matters more, individually or collectively, than our health. Regardless of political allegiance, Canadians are nearly unanimous that a universal health system is a good thing—for reasons of economics and social justice. That's why every Western country save one has a universal system. When it comes to health care, only the United States is morally bankrupt and economically inept.

Canadians take pride in besting the United States on the health front, but it is a hollow victory. In reality, every other developed country has universal health care that is better, fairer and cheaper than ours. We are big on grand pronouncements such as, "Medicare is what defines us as Canadians." But we are laggards on the practical side.

Canadians want care that is appropriate, timely, accessible, safe and affordable, from birth until death. Yet our system is failing on virtually all those measures. Why? For starters, we lack vision and goals. Canadian health care is a $228-billion-a-year enterprise with no clear goals and a dearth of leadership. We talk endlessly about the sustainability of medicare but have no idea what we want to sustain. Our medicare model is a relic, frozen in time. Tommy Douglas's role in shaping publicly funded health insurance for hospital and physician care is celebrated, mythologized even. But we conveniently ignore that medicare was designed to meet the needs of 1950s Canada.

In 1957—when the program became nominally national—the

average age of Canadians was twenty-seven. Health care consisted of acute, episodic care: going to the doctor for treatment of an infectious disease, or to the hospital to give birth, have surgery or die. Today, the average age of Canadians is forty-seven. The technological advances of the past half century have been dizzying. The great majority of our care needs are now for treatment of chronic illnesses. Yet neither the model for delivering care nor the insurance payment model has adapted to the new reality. You can't deliver modern health care with a 1950s model.

So how do we drag medicare, kicking and screaming, into the twenty-first century? Our favoured response has been to throw more bodies and more money at problems. But the solutions need to be more fundamental and come on two levels: funding and delivery.

Let's start with delivery. Action is required in five broad areas:

- *Primary care.* Essentially, we need to take our hospital-based care system and turn it on its head to make community-based primary care the focus. We need to move away from an acute, episodic-care model to a chronic-care model. Every Canadian needs a medical home, a central co-ordination point for their care—preventive, acute and chronic—and an electronic medical record. And care should be delivered by teams, not individual practitioners, due to the complexity.
- *Drugs.* We need to extend universal health coverage to prescription drugs. Currently, through a patchwork of public and private schemes, about thirty-five million Canadians have drug insurance (twenty-four million are covered by private plans and eleven million by public plans, but hundreds of thousands have no drug coverage). A public plan need not pay for everything from Aspirin to Zyprexa, just the essentials. Nor does it have to be a centralized bureaucracy. Quebec has demonstrated that a universal prescription drug program—a mix of public and private insurance—is feasible and affordable.
- *Home care.* We need to treat people where they live, in the community, not in expensive, soulless, germ-ridden institutions.

Too expensive? Not if it's an alternative to hospital and nursing-home care. For example, seventy-five hundred Canadians currently live in hospitals—meaning they have been discharged but have nowhere to go—and that's the tip of the iceberg.

· *Social determinants.* We need to invest in prevention efforts, particularly for socially disadvantaged and marginalized groups such as indigenous people. Let's stop pretending that health is merely a medical issue, and spending as though it were. Good education, housing, income and the environment are essential to good health. A whole-of-government approach is required.

· *Quality.* Safe, prompt and effective must be the guiding principles for care delivery. For the most part, these are engineering and administrative issues, not medical ones. Care is rationed in every country. You can ration by creating financial barriers, as they do in the United States, or you can ration based on results—which ensures everyone gets basic, effective care. Quality care is cheaper in the long run.

Reforming the delivery of care is the easy part. In Canada, funding is unquestionably the Gordian knot.

Spreading risk—and health costs—across the entire population, as we do with medicare, is a good model. But an essential element is missing that undermines medicare: a failure to define clearly what is covered by public insurance and what is not. Canadians have to accept that public-health insurance covers only the basics. At the same time, those who oversee the system have to recognize that physician and hospital care is not enough in the twenty-first century. We need to expand the areas medicare covers—into drugs, home care, long-term care—while at the same time limiting coverage across the board to the essentials.

Universal coverage is not a synonym for unlimited, open-ended coverage. There are choices to be made. They include:

· As stated already, defining clearly what is covered by medicare and what is not.

- Paying only for what works. Many interventions are of dubious value or are not cost-effective. They shouldn't be covered by public insurance.
- Paying a lot more attention to patients with complex needs because they drive costs. One percent of patients account for 25 percent of costs, and 5 percent account for half of all spending.
- Instituting a means test. An equitable system does not mean providing equal services to all at equal cost; user fees and co-payments are not necessarily unfair, but these approaches have to be used smartly.
- Regulating rather than outlawing private insurance and care. One of the most important lessons we should take from Europeans is that we need a combination of a well-regulated private system and a well-managed public system.

The so-called public–private debate is the third rail of Canadian health politics. But it's a false dichotomy. Every health system worth its salt has a mix of private and public delivery and payment. In every country, including this one, most delivery is done by private providers. (That includes not-for-profits, for-profit businesses and independent contractors such as doctors.) On the funding side, the split is usually in the 70:30 to 80:20 range, public–private. The only unique feature of Canadian medicare is the bifurcated payment system. Hospitals and doctors are 100 percent publicly funded. Other services—drugs, home care, long-term care and dental—get between zero and 50 percent public funding.

The question is not whether or not we have private and public care. It's getting the mix right. Private enterprise does certain things well, and public and non-profit enterprises do certain things well. Let's be pragmatic and benefit from both, as most European countries do. We need to pay much more attention to equity—making sure everyone is cared for—and less to who is delivering the services.

Implementing these changes will, of course, require leadership. But nothing is radically new in these proposals. The real challenge in Canadian health care is implementing what we already know is needed. Everyone has a role to play: Ottawa, the provinces and territories, health professionals, allied workers, labour, business, consumer groups, patients and citizens. But they all have to put a little water in their wine—and whine a little less. Reform is going to happen only if the political environment changes, if we stop shouting down every proposal for change because it threatens vested interests. It's time for the interests of patients—and society more broadly—to rule. We don't need a values debate. We don't need more tiresome private–public rhetoric. We don't need Chicken Little screaming that medicare is unsustainable. We need a debate about structure and funding and priorities.

Let's be frank. For many years, we have failed to live up to our responsibilities. We have been lazy and we have been profligate in our spending. But there is reason for optimism. The public isn't just ready for change—the public is demanding it. It's time to stop talking and start acting.

----\|\----

Stop moaning about medicare

I n April of 2005, the *Los Angeles Times* ran a fascinating story about a growing underclass of Americans who have been dubbed the "insured poor." The story is still relevant today. Reporter Daniel Costello told some chilling tales about working stiffs struggling mightily to pay their monthly health-insurance premiums. It was noteworthy that the people profiled—the working poor, middle-class white-collar and blue-collar workers, small business owners—all had stable, long-term employment, yet they were all on the precipice of joining the forty-five million Americans without any health coverage.

There was Terri Matthews, a teacher's aide, who spent US$613 a month for her family's health insurance, one-quarter of her take-home pay. Rather than go without coverage, she skimped on other basics. Matthews stopped heating her home and dropped her car insurance. Ron Dybas owned a lumber company for seventeen years, but he shut it down to take a job with a business that had health benefits because he could no longer afford to pay one-third of his income, US$729 a month, to insure his family. "Such sacrifices for health insurance are far from rare," Costello wrote. "As employees continue to absorb more of their health-care costs, an increasing number of people—even healthy ones—are drastically altering their lives simply to hold on to their insurance. They are delaying home ownership, putting off saving for their children's education, or otherwise sacrificing their financial security to guard against a catastrophic medical bill."

In Canada, we like to moan and groan about our medicare system. The care is never fast enough or good enough. We have too much rationing and not enough choice. The solution that is invariably held out is privatization. Private care, we are told, has no waiting lists and no shortage of physicians, and patients have access to the latest and greatest drugs and technologies. And indeed, that may well be true—for a tiny, well-to-do minority. But for all the problems we have in delivering health care in Canada, embracing a profit-driven health system as the United States has done is not the solution because it does not serve consumers well. For a growing number of Americans, health care—any health care—is increasingly inaccessible and unaffordable. In 2015, the average annual premium for a single person was $6,251, and for a family of four the premium was $17,545. Moreover, insurance rates are soaring and coverage is shrinking. Employers are capping what they spend on health, meaning employees have to absorb all premium increases. Insurers are also tightening the services they will pay for and capping payouts so people with chronic illnesses simply run out of coverage. Since 2005, US health premiums have increased more than 25 percent, and deductibles have soared by 67 percent.

Compare that with Canada, where we take health insurance for granted, to the point where we have developed a deeply rooted sense of entitlement: everybody is entitled to be treated now, or sooner. Everyone is entitled to the most recent, most expensive drug, even if the drug is of dubious or marginal benefit. Everyone is entitled to state-of-the-art techniques and equipment, regardless of cost. If we don't get it, we're going to sue. It has reached the point where politicians and policy-makers dare not say no, lest they be publicly eviscerated. And, oh yes, we think our taxes—taxes that pay for the medicare system—are too high.

Canada's medicare system is not perfect. Far from it. But health-care services in Canada are excellent. The system is cost-efficient—at least compared with the United States. Americans spent just over US$10,000 per capita on health care in 2016, compared with Canadians, who spent C$6,299. Put another way, if we spent at the same rate as Americans, our annual health tab would exceed $340 billion, up from the current $228 billion. Canada's medicare system is also largely accessible and equitable. The care is there when you need it—with very few exceptions—regardless of where you work, where you live, the colour of your skin, and your income. We should be proud that our medicare system makes care affordable to all, but we should not use that as an excuse for its flaws, such as unbearably long wait times.

The predicament of the American "working poor" provides some important perspective. For Canadians, it is unimaginable to spend 25 percent or more of our income on health care. But with the costs of private care and out-of-pocket expenses creeping up, especially for prescription drugs, we can't be too self-righteous. Like the house-rich, cash-poor who stretch their finances to pay for housing, the "insured poor" are barely hanging on to their coverage. "Eventually, many probably will lose the battle, joining the forty-five million Americans without medical coverage," Costello wrote. (That figure is now at twenty-nine million, but will likely jump again if President Donald Trump follows through on his promise to dismantle Obamacare.)

In the United States, routine health matters—the birth of a baby, heart disease, depression, arthritis—can have catastrophic conse-quences. Medical bills are the primary cause of personal bankruptcy, affecting more than two million families a year. Notably, all those affected began with private health insurance but soon exhausted it. Illness can also result in job loss, and along with it health insurance just when it is needed most.

Dr. David Himmelstein, an associate professor of medicine

at Harvard University and the study's lead author, put it this way: "Unless you're Bill Gates, you're just one serious illness away from bankruptcy."

Funding overhaul is needed to cure our ailing hospital system

Hospitals are the cornerstone of our health system. We rush to hospital in emergencies; we go there for life-saving surgery and for treatment of serious illness; and, increasingly, chronic illnesses are managed through hospital-based clinics. Hospitals are also powerful symbols. Most Canadians are born in hospitals, and most still die there. A community without a hospital is viewed as a place without a heart or a soul.

Hospitals are the single biggest expense in our health system. Of the $228 billion Canadians spent on health care in 2016, $66 billion went to hospitals, compared with $36.5 billion for drugs and $34.9 billion for physician services. Yet the public knows surprisingly little about how the nine hundred or so hospitals in this country are administered or funded.

Dr. Brian Day, past president of the Canadian Medical Association, said in 2007 that one of his priorities was to change how hospitals were funded. He decried block funding, the transfer of set budgetary amounts from provincial coffers to individual hospitals. What he wanted to see instead was "patient-focused funding," where the money follows the patients and hospitals are allocated money based on the number of patients treated, the procedures performed and the timeliness of care. While discussing the pros and cons of such an approach can be useful, it's also important to examine the issue of block funding and place it in some context. (Day's vision never did come to pass, but a number of jurisdictions have experimented with variations on patient-focused funding.)

Medicare, a state-administered health insurance program, began because people could not afford hospital care. A heart attack, traumatic injury or complicated childbirth could instantly impoverish a family. When governments began to offer "free" hospital care—beginning with Saskatchewan in 1947, fifteen years before physician services were also covered and medicare was born—hospital budgets were reviewed line by line by provincial health officials. By the late 1960s, this process had become onerous, so hospitals were allocated global budgets. The starting point was the previous year's budget, adjusted for inflation and growth—but almost always with a cap. New programs were funded separately for a few years, then rolled into the global budget. From a government point of view, block funding was very successful because it was an effective way to contain costs. For the past forty years, hospitals' share of spending as a percentage of total health expenditures has fallen steadily.

But the shortcomings of block funding are many. Stated bluntly, hospitals on fixed budgets have a perverse incentive to do less to keep costs down. That's why we have surgical floors shutting down during the holidays despite wait-lists. And block funding is, more often than not, inequitable. It is not responsive to increases in the volume of care; nor does it take into account the characteristics of the patient population. Further, block funding doesn't create incentives for cost-effective care. The result is a constant game of catch-up and hospitals with chronic deficits.

But the rigid, bureaucratic block funding of yore no longer exists. Governments have introduced all manner of programs to supplement core budgets. Increasingly, we are seeing regionalization, which allows more sensible funding of programs regardless of where they are delivered (be it hospitals, long-term care facilities, clinics or the community). Governments are also moving to multi-year budgets for hospitals and adopting incentive programs to reward efficiency and quality care. The goal, ultimately, is to ensure that hospitals that provide comparable services receive comparable funds. Budgets also need to take into account the characteristics of the patient population—meaning that hospitals in low-income areas need more money than those in high-income areas. One of the biggest challenges is having budgets and facilities that keep pace in hospitals in communities with explosive growth, like those in parts of Alberta and Southern Ontario. There is also the thorny issue of what to do with hospitals that underperform; few politicians dare shut down a hospital.

In a health system like Canada's, where 90 percent of funding comes from state coffers, overall budget control must remain with the state. We can probably all agree that, in the twenty-first century, block funding is not the way to do it properly. But we must be careful not to trade one set of problems for another. Performance-based funding, while it would introduce the so-called discipline of the marketplace by having hospitals compete with each other for patients, would also cause widespread carnage. Programs, and even entire hospitals, could shut down. Care could be fragmented. Administrative costs would likely increase and so too would overall costs. And while patients might have more choice, would it be meaningful choice?

Regardless, we should be having the discussion, vigorously and publicly. Hospitals are just too important and too expensive to simply accept the status quo and not strive to do better.

Canada's two-tiered health system: The rural–urban split

Running a health system in a country as vast and sparsely populated as Canada poses many challenges, big and small. But some of those seemingly small challenges have vast implications. Take the case of Flower's Cove, Newfoundland. Located near the tip of the Great Northern Peninsula, the coastal community has a population of about three hundred—and maybe double that number if you include the surrounding areas. Flower's Cove is home to the Strait of Belle Isle Health Centre, which operates twenty-four hours a day, seven days a week. It offers basic emergency services, everyday family medicine (provided largely by nurse practitioners), an ambulance service (principally for transport to larger health-care facilities), home-care nurses, dental care and medical diagnostic services, including some laboratory testing and X-rays.

On August 31, 2009, the provincial government decided to cut back the operating time of the clinic to twelve hours a day and shut down the lab. A great hue and cry followed, with protests in the streets. The health minister, Paul Oram, reversed the decision on the clinic hours so emergency services would again be available around the clock. Then he resigned, saying the non-stop pressure and scrutiny of even the most mundane decisions was taking a toll on his personal health. "There's no end to the stress and strain," Oram said in his words of farewell.

Flower's Cove is, in many ways, representative of the major challenge in our medicare system: Where do we draw the lines? And who draws them? Canadians have developed an incredible sense of medicare entitlement: we want all care for all people, instantly and free of charge—after all, we pay high taxes! While this may be possible—at least theoretically—in densely populated, infrastructure-rich urban centres, distance poses a major challenge in health-care delivery in huge swaths of the country. Canada's land mass is about 95 percent rural/remote, but less than 30 percent of its population lives in rural/remote areas.

In reality, we have a two-tiered health system, but it's not a private–public split, it's an urban–rural split. The health outcomes of those who live in remote settings are poor compared with urban and suburban dwellers: life expectancy is lower, child mortality is higher, injury rates are astronomical and there is far more obesity and chronic illness such as heart disease. Much of this can be explained by the fact that residents of rural communities are poorer and older (with the exception of indigenous communities, which have their own particular health challenges).

The reality, too, is these challenges predate the creation of medicare half a century ago, when the folkloric country doctor trudged miles on foot in a snowstorm to save a patient's life. If anything, the factors that impede the availability of, and access to, good-quality care for rural residents have been exacerbated by technological advances and social change.

The question is, how do you improve the situation? Do you build a twenty-four-hour-a-day health clinic in every community, even those with a few hundred residents? A hospital in slightly larger centres? If so, how do you staff them? Modern medicine is heavily dependent on diagnostic testing. Do you build a lab in every outport? If so, how do you ensure quality and cost-efficiency? What about surgery? Should that be done in small hospitals or only in larger institutions? After all, we know that outcomes are far better in high-volume centres.

We have this jingoistic love for hospitals and health clinics—communities that don't have one or two feel inadequate and neglected. But are patients not better served by having high-quality diagnostic tests done at a central lab and getting the results by e-mail or FedEx than being dependent on a rinky-dink facility? Should scarce health-care dollars not be invested wisely in improving transportation and family support so patients can be treated in well-equipped regional centres with a minimum of disruption instead of dotting the landscape with clinics that overreach their abilities? More important still, can we not have these discussions without their being subsumed by political rhetoric? Can we not make rational, good-for-the-system decisions without them being substituted by politically expedient ones?

The tragedy of Flower's Cove is not whether the clinic lost a lab or some operating hours. In the grand scheme of things that doesn't really matter. What matters is that ten thousand Flower's Coves exist across Canada. Tough decisions need to be made—and a balance found. But decision-makers can seemingly no longer make decisions. Politicians like Paul Oram have become punching bags for those with vested interests. Health administrators and government bureaucrats whose role should be to ensure the delivery of quality care in a cost-effective manner have been emasculated. Anytime their policies make ripples, they get trashed. (And the media do a lot of aiding and abetting.) Is that any way to run a health system?

Here's a radical health-care
idea: Put the patient first

"Our current health system has been designed around the people who deliver the care. It is time to realign the values of the health system so that the patient is again made the centre of attention." That is just one of the refreshingly frank comments found in *For Patients' Sake*, a report out of Saskatchewan, one that should be mandatory reading for every politician, health administrator and health professional.

Patient-centred care and family-centred care are the buzz terms *du jour*. But there is a lot more talk than innovative action. Offering up convenient, timely care, making it easy to navigate the system, actually communicating with patients and treating them with respect do not seem like radical ideas, but sadly, they are far from the norm. There are too many self-interested lobby groups and too many silos, and there is always too little time to listen. Health professionals want to deliver high-quality, compassionate care (and despite the barriers, often do). But they are too beholden to systems and constrained by traditional ways of doing things to put patients and their families first.

Saskatchewan, to its credit, decided to move beyond the rhetoric. In November 2008, health minister Don McMorris announced the Patient First Review, under the leadership of long-time health administrator Tony Dagnone. The health system has had many federal and provincial reviews over the years, so the move was greeted with a lot of eye-rolling and yawns. But the strength of the Patient First Review was that it focused on two key questions:

- Is the health system putting the patient first?
- Is the health system achieving good value in care delivery and system administration?

The other strength was Dagnone himself, a man with a Tommy Douglas–like passion for medicare, coupled with an insider's knowledge of the system's strengths and weaknesses. In the half century since the foundations of medicare were forged out of Prairie populism and the pursuit of social justice, Canada has built an excellent universal, state-funded insurance program. (Or, more precisely, fifteen vaguely interlocking programs, but that is a discussion for another time.) But the underlying theme of Dagnone's report was that, along the way, we lost sight of the people the system was designed to serve: the patients and, by extension, their family members.

What was needed to repair this fundamental flaw, he said, was not more rejigging of bureaucratic structures but a change of culture and a rethinking of priorities. "Patients ask that health-care workers and their respective leadership see beyond their declared interests so that the interest of patients takes precedence at every care interaction, every future contract negotiation and every policy debate," Dagnone wrote. "Only in this way will we achieve a patient- and family-centred health system for Saskatchewan citizens. Similarly, government leaders and policy-makers must keep the patient front and centre when policies, programs and new models of care are designed and implemented."

The formulation of that statement is noteworthy. "Patients ask" is used because the commissioner did extensive consultations with patients and families. Dagnone did what is so rarely done in the day-to-day operations of the health system: he asked patients what they wanted and then he actually listened to them. A vast reservoir of untapped patient knowledge exists that we need to explore to improve medicare. What the commissioner heard is that the system performs relatively well. The care is good, but not good enough.

So where does medicare fall down on the job? In a few areas:

· *Convenience and timeliness.* There is too much waiting, and it's not easy to get in the right door for care, so people end up in emergency rooms by default.
· *Lack of co-ordination.* Patients do not move seamlessly through

the system; there are often big cracks to fall through at transfer points.
- *Lack of equitable care.* Patients want reasonable access to care but feel they are discriminated against based on where they live, their age, their ethnicity and other factors.
- *Lack of communication and information.* When someone is sick or injured, they are frightened. They crave basic information, but everyone is too busy.
- *Lack of electronic health records.* Patients hate repeating their medical histories over and over, and tests are oft-repeated because of lack of modern records.
- *Lack of respect.* All too often, patients feel they are treated as a bother to health professionals. Patients are not cost centres, they are the raison d'être of the system.

Dagnone does not use the term, but reading his report one is left with the sense that the primary frustration with medicare is the total lack of customer service. That does not seem like an insurmountable barrier. In fact, Dagnone concludes that there is no need to dismantle and reinvent the health system but rather the need for a collective will and vision to implement fixes and change the culture of caring. "'Patient First' must become more than a mantra. For the sake of patients it must become a movement that is embraced by all who have a stake in creating healthier communities."

—⋀—

Montreal's super-hospital saga was a historic farce

It took twenty-two years in the early seventeenth century to build the Taj Mahal, the awe-inspiring white marble mausoleum in Agra, India. It took longer than that for Quebec to build a utilitarian hospital in Montreal in the twenty-first century.

The Taj Mahal is a glowing symbol of eternal love. The "Taj Hôpital" is a shameful symbol of political dithering. In a December 2010 instalment of the absurdist tale, then-Quebec Treasury Board president Michelle Courchesne announced that construction of the Centre hospitalier de l'Université de Montréal (CHUM) would begin the following spring and be completed by 2019. The tentative price: $2.1 billion. Well, she actually announced that there would eventually be another announcement because bids had yet to be tendered. Not to mention there were no final blueprints. And so it went.

The idea of building a Montreal "super-hospital"—merging archaic institutions scattered around the city into one state-of-the-art facility—was first floated in 1991. It was an eminently wise plan, particularly in a city where most health-care facilities were built decades and in some cases centuries ago. But in the health field there is no idea, however sensible, that cannot be bogged down by bureaucracy and perverted by politics. The Quebec super-hospital saga is a case in point. (In the interest of brevity, let's leave out names and political affiliations: suffice it to say that six premiers and ten ministers of health have been involved in the file to date, and the Liberals and Péquistes have handled it in equally bumbling style.)

In 1995, Quebec's health minister announced a merger of the three "French" hospitals—Hôtel-Dieu, Notre-Dame and Saint-Luc—to create CHUM. A similar process happened with the "English" hospitals—Montreal General, Royal Victoria, Montreal Chest Institute, Montreal Neurological Hospital and Lachine Hospital—and that was called the McGill University Health Centre (MUHC). In 1999, it was finally decided that CHUM and MUHC should be more than virtual institutions. They would become bricks-and-mortar "super-hospitals."

Then the real jockeying began. Where would the facilities be built? What would happen with the existing hospital properties? How many beds would each super-hospital have? And so on. Forests were felled and tens of millions of dollars spent to produce studies, including a 2003 commission of inquiry headed by former prime minister Brian Mulroney and former Quebec premier Daniel Johnson.

Back then, CHUM was going to cost $860 million, and the super-hospitals were going to be built and operating by 2007. But a shovel in the ground by this date would prove to be a pipe dream. One of the most politically vicious battles was about the future site of CHUM. It came down to 1000 St-Denis St. (in the heart of downtown) or 6000 St-Denis St. (in tony Outremont). There is enough intrigue in those choices to fill a book—and, in fact, a book has been written. The travails of MUHC, by contrast, were minor. All they had to deal with was contaminated land and angry neighbours near the planned construction site in Notre-Dame-de-Grâce. And, oh yes, the costly foot-dragging of indecisive political leaders and a kickback scandal.

Plans to have the new facilities built as private–public partnerships (PPPs)—an approach in which private enterprise would build the hospitals, then lease them back to government over a thirty-year period—added to the controversy and cost and, in the end, private enterprise would play a token financing role so the government could save face. By 2016, the 772-bed CHUM's projected total cost was $2.1 billion, along with a $470 million CHUM research centre. Not to mention the $500 million upgrade of Sainte-Justine, the "French" pediatric hospital. MUHC cost about $2.4 billion, including a new five-hundred-bed facility, a new Montreal Children's Hospital and extensive renovations to the 332-bed Montreal General Hospital. That's $5.5 billion and counting—though one economist calculated that when the final tally is in, the total will reach $8.6 billion.

That sort of profligate spending is difficult to justify, but the fact remains that all the facilities were needed and overdue. Quebec's flagship hospitals were crumbling, inefficient and increasingly unsafe. (It's no coincidence that Quebec had an inordinate number of hospital-acquired infections such as *C. difficile*.) Quebec's political leaders should have received credit for their bold investments in health care. Instead, they received derision because they took too long to do the right thing. They lost sight of who really matters: the public. An endless list of excuses was trotted out each time a minister made a new announcement and revised the timeline for construction. But the bottom line is that these hospitals should have been up and running at the turn of the new millennium. The delays served the interests of property developers, construction companies, donors to political parties and various interest groups within the health system, not the sick and injured who needed hospital care.

Almost two and a half decades after planning began, the MUHC finally opened in April of 2015, while the CHUM is slated to open sometime in 2017. That no premier or health minister ever demanded that the shuffling of paper end and the roar of construction equipment begin is a disgrace, plain and simple. In Canada, we talk a good game about patient-centred care. But it will never be a reality unless it becomes a priority and a guiding principle from the upper echelons of power on down.

When even Dr. Optimism is losing faith in medicare, it's time to fix it

"We have seen a slow and steady decline in what we would all now agree is a deeply troubled health-care system. To be clear, this pillar of Canadian society is eroding ... We are losing something of great value. It's slipping away slowly, incrementally."

This kind of rhetoric is so commonplace that we have become largely inured to it. At first blush, it's another medicare-is-doomed pronouncement much as we've heard seemingly every day for the past half century or so. But pay attention this time—those mournful words were spoken by Dr. Jeffrey Turnbull, past president of the Canadian Medical Association, in his valedictory address of August 2011.

Turnbull is one of the most unwaveringly hopeful and positive people in medicine. He knows the Canadian health system inside out, and from the bottom up. He cheerfully treats poor, homeless addicts as part of Ottawa's Inner City Health project. He is equally upbeat as chief of staff at the Ottawa Hospital, a thankless position. He affably headed the CMA, which speaks and lobbies on behalf of the single most powerful and prickly group in the health system, physicians.

If Turnbull is losing faith in medicare, we need to prick up our ears—and roll up our sleeves and fix it. When he expresses his frustration, it is not rhetoric. He backs his feelings with cold, hard facts and incisive anecdotes. "I've always been immensely proud of our health-care system—one that was once considered to be one of the best in the world," he told CMA delegates. "But times have changed and Canada now ranks below Slovenia in terms of effectiveness and last or second last in terms of value for money." Ouch. Equally scathing is his summary of the frustrations he has heard expressed by patients in his travels coast to coast. "They've told us they're suffering because of a lack of access to timely, effective care, confused by a system that is limited in the services it provides, that is cumbersome and almost too complex to navigate, and angered by a system that fails to put their needs first or even engage them about their health issues."

That takes care of the international comparisons and shortcomings in care delivery. What about administration of the $228-billion-a-year health system? "I've been struck by the lack of leadership, co-ordinated management, accountability, and responsibility—and, yes, needless waste," Turnbull said. "Worse, we allow staggering inefficiency, ineffective management processes, incoherent decision-making and practice variations that undermine quality and safety." Despite it all, he remains optimistic. "I do believe this can be changed ... that we can create a better health-care system in the future."

Turnbull has a diagnosis and a prescription. It begins with getting back to basics. Medicare—and other social programs—were created to address social inequities, to make good health achievable and affordable for all. Yet today in Canada there is "devastating and epidemic health inequity"—and it has become a major driver of health costs. One way to address inequality in health-care delivery is to ensure all Canadians have access to a basic level of prescription-drug coverage, a "glaring failure" of medicare, Turnbull said. Similarly, there needs to be a massive shift in approach (and resources), from the 1950s-style illness-care system we have now to a twenty-first-century health system that emphasizes chronic care and prevention.

In his time as CMA president, Turnbull championed this transformation. He created a blueprint, a document titled *Health Care Transformation in Canada: Change That Works, Care That Lasts*. It's by no means perfect, but it's a start. It does not merely advocate shoring up the system that is eroding but rebuilding it from the ground up—all the while keeping the foundation, the public insurance model. As Turnbull told his CMA colleagues, "Leadership demands vision to see the path before us, the courage to take it and the strength to follow it." Not just hope, not just words, but purposeful actions.

———⊣⊢———

Is Canada's public health-care system financially unsustainable?

I t is often stated that Canada's health system is *unsustainable*—a vague, undefined term that is used as a synonym for unafford-able. The problem is the unsustainability argument is based on a few dubious assumptions:

- that annual spending will continue to grow at the same rate as in the past, if not faster;
- that the aging of the population will actually accelerate the spending increases; and
- that nothing can be done to reduce spending. This, in turn, assumes that nothing can be done to change the way we deliver health care or to keep people healthier longer.

In short, it is a pretty cynical world view. And, more importantly, concrete solutions are rarely proposed to alleviate the problem, other than to privatize more health services. Philosophical arguments aside, doing so does not reduce overall costs but merely shifts them from the collectivity to individuals, from public insurance plans to private ones or, worse yet, to out-of-pocket costs. What this dreary set of assumptions does do, however, is remind us of one of the major failings of Canada's publicly funded health system: we do very little planning and analysis, especially of a financial nature. That's why a 2013 report from the Canadian Institute of Actuaries was a welcome contribution, albeit a modest one.

The CIA (the actuaries, not the US spy agency) undertook a straightforward task: to create a model for projecting future health-care costs. They chose the province of New Brunswick as an example of how that model could be used. The limitation was that the modelling exercise examined only steady-state health-care costs—meaning costs based on the assumption that there would be no changes to health-care coverage or financing, and no major changes in the economic environment. But this was nonetheless useful because it provided some concrete data about what health spending would look like if all things remained the same. In this analysis, health costs were predicted to rise 4.43 percent annually until 2020, just as they had done in the previous decade. Practically, that meant the provincial health budget would increase to $4.6 billion in 2020 from $2.8 billion in 2009. Per-capita costs would rise to $5,976 from $3,711 in that same period. Put another way, at the time of the study it cost about $75 a week to provide health care to each of the 750,000 residents of New Brunswick. By 2020, it will cost $115 a week. (That is slightly above the Canadian average.)

Is that unreasonable? Unsustainable? The actuaries' report didn't answer those questions. It just crunched the numbers. But data make for a much more concrete discussion than rhetoric.

One of the more interesting sets of numbers was a breakdown of the 4.43 percent annual increase. Based on data from the Canadian Institute for Health Information, the actuaries said the rise in health costs had three main elements:

· Health-care inflation accounted for 1.99 percent of the increase, money that goes mostly to wage increases. In fact, about two-thirds of all health spending is for labour.

- Aging, which is often cited—wrongly—as the principal reason health costs are becoming unsustainable, accounted for 1.27 percent of the annual rise in costs. This is because per-capita costs increase as people age.
- Increased utilization made up the rest of the cost escalation, at 1.10 percent. This is a reminder that people of all ages are using more services, not just seniors.

The report also estimated projected annual increases in major categories, including hospitals, physician services, drugs and other institutions (like nursing homes). Overall, the numbers are sobering. Without changes in how we deliver health care, per-capita costs will have tripled from 2000 to 2020: to $3,599 from $1,219 for hospitals; $1,105 from $354 for physicians; and $452 from $104 for drugs.

These data give some ammunition to those who argue that the system is unsustainable, at least superficially. But what they should really do is provide impetus for reform. Canadians don't need a discussion of how to rein in costs, because that usually results in little more than trimming around the edges. What we need to discuss is delivering care differently, including actuarial modelling of new approaches.

A public insurance plan should, like a private plan, ensure that it has enough money to provide insured services. But the first crucial step is determining what those insured services are. Those are political and societal choices. The accounting exercise comes later.

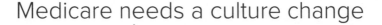

Medicare needs a culture change

"Canada is a country of perpetual pilot projects," Monique Bégin famously wrote in the *Canadian Medical Association Journal*. The former minister of health and welfare pithily described a long-standing, frustrating problem in our medicare system: we have solved every single problem in our health-care system ten times over, but we seem incapable of scaling up the solutions.

This inability to learn, to share and embrace innovation across jurisdictions, is explored thoughtfully in the 2015 report of the Advisory Panel on Healthcare Innovation. The panel, led by David Naylor, a physician and former president of the University of Toronto, emphasized that "Canada has no shortage of innovative health-care thinkers, world-class health researchers, capable executives, or dynamic entrepreneurs who see opportunity in the health sphere." But innovation is stifled by the structure and administration of the health system, and by a dearth of leadership. Medicare—the name we give our publicly funded health-insurance scheme—is, in fact, not a system at all; it's a collection of fourteen federal, provincial and territorial programs (plus Workers' Compensation, which is private) that are neither integrated nor co-ordinated. Worse yet, within those programs, there is a near total absence of vision and goals.

The role of our health bureaucrats is to hold the line on spending as best they can and, above all, ensure that the names of their political masters don't appear in damaging headlines. Improving patient care is rarely the number-one priority. The way our system is funded—predominantly with block transfers to hospitals and fee-for-service payments to physicians—encourages volume of procedures and the status quo. It does not reward quality of care or responsible stewardship. In fact, when an individual or a program goes out on a limb and makes changes to improve efficiency or cost-effectiveness, the benefits often accrue to others; perverse disincentives are commonplace and counterproductive.

These problems and frustrations are not new. The Naylor report cites an example from 1974, when Canadian researchers published a landmark paper showing that nurse practitioners could do 70 percent of doctors' work with no difference in outcomes or patient satisfaction. Using nurse practitioners also saved money, but hiring more of them was hampered by the fact that, generally speaking, doctors are paid on a fee-for-service basis and nurses are salaried. Over four decades later, that same bureaucratic hurdle remains. Most other Western countries acted on the research: nurse practitioners are an integral part of health-care delivery and most physicians are salaried. But in Canada, nurse practitioners are still grossly underused—except in pilot projects, of course. We still negotiate physician and nurse contracts separately, and our management of health-care human resources is a mess. Until you get workers with the right skills in the right place at the right time, you will never deliver seamless, patient-centred care and you will never control costs, because labour accounts for two-thirds of all spending. As the nurse practitioner story and countless not-acted-upon research findings have since illustrated, innovation is hampered by policy gridlock. The managers of the system are largely powerless and beholden to the whims of politicians; moreover, with few exceptions, they are profoundly mistrusting of entrepreneurship and pathologically risk-averse.

For decades, we have produced reports about the need to transform health-care delivery and funding while simultaneously clinging to the same old way of doing things. It's a fundamental disconnect between evidence and action. If you don't take risks, you will never innovate. So how do we break the log-jam? According to the Naylor report, it has to begin with leadership, and it should come from Ottawa.

One of the panel's central recommendations is the creation of an independent health innovation agency to not just fund pilot projects but to promote scaling up, to use searchable repositories of successful programs, to offer financial incentives and to encourage regulatory change—all with the aim of spurring innovation. More resources alone will not ensure the scaling up of good ideas. There needs to be partnership, commitment and monitoring to ensure implementation. In short, it's not more money the system needs, it's culture change—a shift from perpetual pilot projects to embracing innovation and best practices.

Canada needs a "coalition of the willing" to fix health care

Which country has the world's best health system? That is one of those unanswerable questions that health-policy geeks like to ponder and debate, and serious attempts have been made at measuring and ranking. In 2000, the World Health Organization (in)famously produced a report that concluded that France had the world's best health system, followed by those of Italy, San Marino, Andorra and Malta. The business publication *Bloomberg* produces an annual ranking that emphasizes value for money from health spending; the 2015 ranking placed Singapore on top, followed by Hong Kong, Spain, South Korea, Japan and Italy. The Economist Intelligence Unit compares 166 countries and ranks Japan as number one, followed by Singapore, Switzerland, Iceland and Australia. The Commonwealth Fund ranks health care in eleven Western countries and gives the nod to the United Kingdom, followed by Switzerland, Sweden, Australia and Germany.

The problem with these exercises is that no one can really agree on what should be measured and, even when they do settle on measures, data are not always reliable and comparable. "Of course, there is no such thing as a perfect health system and it certainly doesn't reside in any one country," Mark Britnell, global chairman for health at the consulting giant KPMG, writes in his book, *In Search of the Perfect Health System* (Palgrave Macmillan, 2015). "But there are fantastic examples of great health and health care from around the world which can offer inspiration."

As a consultant who has worked in sixty countries—and who receives in-depth briefings on the health systems of each before meeting clients—Britnell has a unique perspective and, in his book, offers up a subjective and insightful list of the traits that are important to creating good health systems. If the world had a perfect health system, he writes, it would have the following qualities: the values and universal access of the United Kingdom; the primary care of Israel; the community services of Brazil; the mental-health system of Australia; the health promotion philosophy of the Nordic countries; the patient and community empowerment in parts of Africa; the research and development infrastructure of the United States; the innovation, flair and speed of India; the information, communications and technology of Singapore; the choice offered to patients in France; the funding model of Switzerland; and the care for the aged of Japan.

In his book, Britnell elaborates on each of these examples of excellence; in addition, he provides a great précis of the strengths and weaknesses of health systems in twenty-five countries. The chapter on Canada is appropriately damning, noting that this country's outmoded health system has long been ripe for revolution, but the "revolution has not happened." Why? Because this country has a penchant for doing high-level, in-depth reviews of the health system's problems, but puts all its effort into producing recommendations and none into implementing them. "Canada stands at a crossroads," Britnell writes, "and needs to find the political will and managerial and clinical skills to establish a progressive coalition of the willing."

The book's strength is that it does not offer up simplistic solutions. Rather, it stresses that there is no single best approach because all health systems are the products of their societies, norms and cultures. One of the best parts of the book—and quite relevant to Canada—is the analysis of funding models. "The debate about universal health care is frequently confused with the ability to pay," Britnell writes. He notes that the high co-payments in the highly praised health systems of Asia would simply not be tolerated in the West.

But ultimately, what matters is finding not a perfect approach but one that works: "This is the fundamental point. There is no such thing as free health care; it is only a matter of who pays for it. Politics is the imperfect art of deciding 'who gets what, how and when.'" The book stresses that the challenges are the same everywhere: providing high-quality care to all at an affordable price, finding the workforce to deliver that care, and empowering patients. To do so effectively, we need vision and we need systems. Above all, we need the political will to learn from others and put in place a system that works.

——∿——

Taking patient-centred care
from rhetoric to reality

Patient-centred care is a term that gets bandied about a lot these days. But what does it really mean? How does our health system need to change to make it truly patient-centred? What reforms and innovations are required on a systems level? How do front-line care providers need to change to make care truly patient centred? And how do patients need to behave differently? These are all questions that need to be answered if we're going to move from feel-good rhetoric to doing-some-good reality.

The US Health and Medicine Division of the National Academies of Sciences, Engineering, and Medicine defines patient-centred care as "care that is respectful and responsive to individual patient preferences, needs and values." That's nice and inspiring and all-encompassing. It means everything and nothing. There's a well-worn expression: "I don't know anything about art, but I know what I like." Patient-centred care is a bit like that; you know when you experience it—and especially when you don't—but you can't necessarily articulate the characteristics.

In many ways, the concept is more easily expressed in aphorisms than with a formal definition. "The needs of the patient come first" is the tagline of the Mayo Clinic; "Every patient is the only patient" was carved above the front entrance of the Harvard Community Health Plan Hospital. "Nothing about me without me" is the rallying cry of many patient activists. Another description of patient-centred care is a more esoteric one: "Giving a patient a better day." When all is said and done, that's what health care is all about: making patients feel a bit better. But like many aspirational goals in health care, these things tend to be a lot easier to say than to do, a lot easier to promise than to deliver. Maybe a better way to understand what patient-centred care means is to articulate what it is and isn't.

So what do patients dislike about being in the health system—aside from being sick, of course? A number of things: the helplessness, the feeling of anonymity, the discontinuity of care, the rote and repetition, being talked about and talked to rather than talked with, the waiting, and the loneliness. Judith John, a long-time health-care executive who was diagnosed with an inoperable brain tumour sixteen years ago, has, along the way, become an eloquent and inspiring patient advocate. She says that in a system that has become obsessed with data, with measuring and metrics, we often lose sight of the importance of relationships, conversation and, ultimately, the person. "When you're a patient, there's only one metric that matters," she says. "Treat me like a person. Not a chart, not a number, but a person."

The failure to do so, which generates so much angst and fear, stems from a fragmented system and from poor communication. We have a sprawling, elaborate, expensive health system with buildings and equipment and all manner of health professionals, but we haven't quite figured out where the patient fits in. There is a broad range of views on this—a spectrum that ranges from radical consumerism, a belief that the patient is God (or, if you prefer, the customer is always right), through to classic professionalism (or, more accurately, paternalism), which holds that medical professionals have to use their knowledge to give patients what is best for them and, in many cases, to protect them from themselves.

Let's not forget the etymology of the word *patient*. It means "to suffer," or more precisely, to be silent in your suffering. Perhaps we need a new word. At the very least, we could use a new definition. Patient-centredness has come to mean "empowerment." But it does not—or should not—mean giving patients everything they want, when they want it. Health care is not an all-you-can-eat Chinese buffet. But it's not a military exercise either, where patients must unquestioningly follow orders. In between those two extremes is the sweet spot: partnership, sharing of information, exchange of opinions, mutual respect. These are all the characteristics you want to see in a patient–provider relationship—and in the system–patient relationship, for that matter.

While these ideals sound great on paper, they are not easy to achieve, especially in the high-octane daily grind that is modern medicine. A whole academic literature exists on shared decision-making and its complexity. Health-care providers need to act in the best interests of patients. But patients often have a view of what is best for them that differs radically from the guidelines and medical teachings. Shared decision-making is about more than agreeing to disagree: it's a lot dirtier and messier than that. It's about finding a compromise that respects medical responsibility and patient autonomy. It's a delicate dance that we're going to have to master if we truly want quality, patient-centred, appropriate care.

----/\----

Lack of dental-care insurance is a gaping hole in medicare

Canada's medicare system has many quirks, but one of the more glaring anomalies is that the mouth does not seem to be considered a part of the body. In our predominantly publicly funded and publicly delivered health system, almost all dental care is funded privately, through employer-based insurance or out-of-pocket. The result is that many Canadians—about one in four—are unable to access dental care. The most vulnerable are the hardest hit. "The system is really not working, and it's only going to get worse unless we act," said Dr. Paul Allison, dean of the faculty of dentistry at McGill University in Montreal.

Annual spending on dental care in Canada tops $13 billion, but only about $800 million of that total is publicly funded. First Nations and Inuit have state-funded dental insurance, at least in theory, but they often have trouble accessing care because they live in remote communities and dentists visit infrequently. Dental care is free for children under ten in Quebec and for those under fourteen in Nova Scotia. All provinces and territories also pay for in-hospital dental surgery—which usually becomes necessary when oral-health problems are neglected for long periods. And a number of ad hoc and charitable programs provide dental care to the poor, many of them run out of Canada's ten schools of dentistry. "But these programs are a drop in the bucket compared to what's needed," Allison said.

Providing "free" dental care to all Canadians under the umbrella of medicare—sometimes referred to as "denticare"—is probably unrealistic in the current economic and political environment. But Allison said there is no question that publicly funded dental-care programs need to be broader and more coherent. They need to provide essential oral care to those most in need, including children in low-income families, seniors living in institutional care, people with disabilities, the homeless, refugees and immigrants, indigenous peoples and those on social assistance.

Why does that matter? Oral diseases, including cavities (which are caused by bacterial infection, not sugar), gingivitis and mouth and tongue cancers, can have a significant impact on daily functioning and quality of life. Dental problems are not merely a nuisance. Evidence is mounting that poor oral health is a bellwether for the rest of the body.

Gum diseases like gingivitis are low-grade infections that cause swelling and bleeding of the gums. The same kind of immune response is triggered as when the immune system fights off bacteria and viruses elsewhere in the body, and this inflammation, particularly in places like the arteries, can have serious consequences, such as exacerbating the symptoms of heart disease or diabetes. Numerous epidemiological studies, including a long-term study of US veterans, show that people with gum disease are far more likely to have heart attacks and strokes. Pregnant women with gum disease are far more likely to have premature and low-birth-weight babies. Diabetics with poor oral health have more symptoms. And some scientists think rotten teeth may even be a factor in cancers; after all, the bacterium *H. pylori*, which causes ulcers, is a key factor in stomach cancer.

Good oral health is clearly not strictly an issue of vanity. Potentially important public-health implications could be derived from better dental care. Healthy habits could ultimately prove to be cheap and effective prevention measures for a host of serious chronic diseases. Yet Canada has one of the lowest rates of publicly funded dental care in the world—only 6 percent of total spending. Even the United States has a higher public share, at 7.9 percent. Many European countries include dental care in their universal health programs. In Finland, for example, 79 percent of dental care is publicly funded.

Dr. Stephen Hwang, a research scientist at the Centre for Research on Inner City Health and a physician at St. Michael's Hospital in Toronto, said lack of dental care is a "gaping hole" in Canadian medicare and causes significant health problems for many of his patients. "Their teeth are atrocious," he said, and the result is that they live in pain, and it affects their nutrition, mental health and cardiovascular health. "These patients have abscesses in their mouths that, if they were in any other part of the body, we would treat," and that's illogical and a false economy because it exacerbates other conditions. "I'm not talking about cosmetics but necessary medical care," Hwang said. "A lot of people aren't getting that necessary care because they can't afford it."

If we want a healthier population—and a more equitable medicare system—we have to put some of our money where our mouths are.

CHAPTER 2

Mental Health

If they are sick, why do we jail the mentally ill?

I magine for a moment that one of the symptoms of breast cancer was an uncontrollable desire to scream obscenities and utter death threats to passersby, or if people with heart disease were prone to masturbating in public, or if those with arthritis developed a compulsion to shoplift. What would we do? Build new women's prisons to ensure breast-cancer sufferers were punished for their transgressions? Construct new sex-offender wings to make room for the legions of people with cardiovascular disease? Jail every arthritic kleptomaniac until they smartened up? Of course, we would never dream of filling jails with people who are already suffering from debilitating but treatable illnesses. Yet that is precisely what we are doing with far too many individuals suffering from mental illnesses including schizophrenia, bipolar disorder and addiction.

Canada has twenty-five thousand criminal offenders incarcerated in provincial and territorial jails and another fifteen thousand in federal penitentiaries, not to mention another hundred thousand under supervision like parole. Of those sentenced to a federal penitentiary (meaning sentences of two years or more), one in four has a diagnosed mental illness, and 80 percent have a serious substance-abuse problem. Federal penitentiaries and provincial jails (as well as our streets) have become de facto mental institutions.

While people with psychiatric conditions can commit criminal acts—as can anyone—many offenders are not responsible for their acts, so they don't belong in prison in the first place. And virtually none of the convicts, whether deserving of prison or not, are getting the treatment they need. In custody, people suffering from mental illness are easy targets; they are vulnerable and exploited. The very behaviours that get people with mental illnesses into trouble in the first place—being loud and belligerent, refusing orders, committing antisocial acts, self-mutilating—make them disciplinary problems. They are sent to solitary confinement, which can exacerbate their symptoms. When they are released, without counselling or assistance, they are virtually doomed to reoffend; thus they are trapped a vicious cycle.

During his tenure as correctional investigator of Canada from 2004 to 2016, Howard Sapers noted repeatedly that care for the mentally ill in prisons is abysmal. Their rights are routinely violated and dignity denied. There is no question the warehousing of the mentally ill in prisons has to end. But for that to happen, we have to address why they end up there in the first place. In modern, progressive Canada, the tool we employ for dealing with the mentally ill is too often the Criminal Code rather than the Mental Health Act.

For almost three decades, provinces have had policies of deinstitutionalization, vowing to liberate the many lifelong patients of institutions for the mentally ill. In the early 1970s, Canada had almost fifty thousand psychiatric beds. Today, there is less than one-tenth of that number. Deinstitutionalization was—and remains—a laudable approach. But implicit in the deal was that care must be provided in the community. Too often, that did not happen. Psychiatric patients were not released into community care, they were just released. This has created an underclass of homeless and semi-homeless "crazy" people who have become fixtures on our streets, and in our jails.

Contrary to stereotypes, most people with mental illness are not violent (except perhaps to themselves). They are eleven times more likely to be victims of violence than perpetrators of violence. For the most part, they are being swept up in the criminal justice system for egregious crimes including public urination, disturbing the peace, vandalism and drunken fights.

You can't blame police. They are armed with guns, batons, handcuffs and the Criminal Code. There is a bit of folk wisdom that holds, "Give a man a hammer and everything becomes a nail." Instead, ideally, police should try to "de-escalate" situations with words rather than brute force. Talk. Wait. Talk some more. But that's not how they are trained or equipped. Invariably, when confronted with people who are unruly, addicted or psychotic, the batons come out; so do the pepper spray, the Taser and sometimes the service revolver. When we invest in weaponry instead of care, tragedy ensues.

Judges, too, have limited options. Some attempts are made at diversion, such as the Mental Health Courts, and judges have the power to order psychiatric evaluations. But with so little assessment capacity and so few beds available, people languish for months in prison waiting for the powers that be to determine whether they should be in the prison system. Courts have already ruled that this practice is illegal and unconstitutional, but it persists.

We don't need a return of Dickensian mental institutions to hide away the "crazies." We need a commitment to integration, to making people with psychiatric illnesses full citizens, with all the rights of citizenship. Deinstitutionalization should not be synonymous with criminalization. We cannot accept that people should be punished for being ill—and mental illness is no exception.

—⎯⫫⎯—

Roofs are needed to patch
the mental-health system

The May 2006 Senate committee report titled *Out of the Shadows at Last: Transforming Mental Health, Mental Illness and Addiction Services in Canada* got a lot of media attention because of one of its quirky recommendations—a nickel-a-drink tax on alcoholic beverages to fund a transformation of the mental-health system. Unfortunately, the focus on this tax proposal detracted attention from a host of excellent and forward-looking recommendations, including an employment program to help people with mental illness land and hold jobs, a call to change employment insurance rules so those suffering from mental illness could qualify more easily, the creation of a mental-health commission, and a large-scale anti-stigma campaign designed to change public attitudes about the mentally ill.

But the most striking and important aspect of the committee's work—led by senators Michael Kirby and Wilbert Keon—was its emphasis on housing. The report made it clear that investing in housing is key to transforming the mental-health system and, more generally, to improving the health of Canadians. Housing is a fundamental determinant of health. You cannot get healthy, or stay healthy, if you do not have a roof over your head. Yet homelessness is all too pervasive in Canada. As the Most Reverend Andrew Hutchison, primate of the Anglican Church of Canada, noted in a commentary piece, "Canada is a rich country. Yet tens of thousands of people live on the street, and millions are without affordable and adequate housing." The homeless are not merely those familiar figures panhandling on street corners or sleeping on grates. The vast majority of the homeless—or perhaps more accurately, the precariously housed—are bunking with friends or family, living in shelters, squatting in abandoned buildings, hanging out in all-night coffee shops, or spending virtually every penny for a bed in a dank welfare hotel. The ranks of the homeless are as diverse as larger society—a mix of young and old, families with children, couples and single people. What they have in common is poverty.

That poverty is the result of any number of underlying causes, the most common being mental-health problems and/or addiction to alcohol or drugs. The Kirby report estimated, conservatively, that at least 140,000 Canadians who are suffering from mental illness have inadequate housing. (The Canadian Mental Health Association says that number may be as high as 300,000.) In addition to those with mental illnesses, there are as many again who are homeless because of physical ailments, unemployment (or, for the working poor, insufficient income from employment), physical or sexual abuse, addiction to alcohol or drugs, a criminal record, or any combination of the above.

It can be a vicious cycle. When a person is precariously housed, their health is poor and their health prospects poorer still. When you are one paycheque or one unexpected expense away from the street, life can quickly spiral downward.

In Canada, we have a terrible habit of tiptoeing around the problem of homelessness. We build soup kitchens and food banks to feed the homeless; we create needle exchanges for intravenous drug addicts; we provide blankets and sleeping bags to street people and even tend to their pets; we build "emergency" shelters and put homeless people up in motels; and we churn the homeless in and out of hospital emergency rooms at tremendous expense. But for all the dollars spent, we invest very little in providing what is really needed—affordable, permanent housing. Doing so—with co-ops, subsidized rent, low-cost mortgages and other measures—should be a fundamental aspect of Canada's social safety net. The failure to provide affordable housing to those in need shows on our streets. Major cities like New York, London and Stockholm do not have the hordes of homeless beggars we see in Toronto, Montreal and Vancouver. That's because they have focused on permanent housing rather than stop-gap measures.

In the past two decades, rental housing construction in Canada has fallen by half, and since 2006, the absolute number of rental properties has steadily declined. The real estate boom is fuelling the rapid destruction of cheap apartments and rooming houses that kept many on the margins off the streets. For its part, the federal government has invested more than $2 billion a year for affordable housing, but as housing prices soar in large cities like Vancouver and Toronto, that seems like a drop in the bucket. Another problem is that the provinces will not (they say *cannot*) provide matching funds. And the Canada Mortgage and Housing Corporation, which is supposed to help Canadians buy homes, turned a $1.4 billion profit in 2015, so it has a lot of wiggle room.

The only solution to homelessness is housing. It's time for Canada to get building—both affordable homes and better health.

Fund suicide prevention,

not metal detectors

T he shooting rampage on September 13, 2006, at Dawson College in Montreal stirred many emotions—chief among them fear, anger and sadness. The death at gunpoint of one teenager, the bullet wounds suffered by a dozen others, the sundry injuries that occurred in the ensuing chaos, the psychological scars that emerged in the aftermath, not to mention the suicide of the killer, should lead us to ponder the broader issues of injury and violence. While much of the discussion in the wake of the Dawson incident focused on gun control and beefing up school security, violence is not merely a criminal issue, nor can dealing with it be the exclusive province of the police, the courts and the penal system.

Violence is a major, and largely neglected, public-health issue. Each year, more than 1.6 million people worldwide die in violent circumstances and many times more are wounded, according to the World Health Organization's most recent data. Of that total, an estimated 815,000 died by suicide, 520,000 were victims of homicide and 310,000 died in armed conflicts, including terrorist attacks. In other words, for all the news headlines about war, murder, suicide bombings and bloody mayhem, the stark reality is that most violence is self-inflicted. In Canada, the statistics show an even greater disparity—more than six suicides for every homicide. Each year, in a country of thirty-six million, we have about six hundred homicides and thirty-nine hundred suicides.

The homicides—particularly the gruesomely public ones such as the death of Anastasia De Sousa at Dawson College—get blanket media coverage. Countless stories and earnest commentaries question what can be done about such senseless violence. The questions are legitimate, but perspective is often lacking. In reality, until middle age, the leading killer in Canada is injuries—from motor vehicle crashes, falls, drownings, violence and suicides. (Worldwide, injuries claim a staggering five million lives annually.)

Most injuries, including most violent deaths, are preventable. That is especially true of suicide. We cannot content ourselves with mopping up the blood, patching the wounds and mending the broken hearts. We need to invest more in the prevention of violence and injuries, but it is not as simple as increasing police presence or adding another course to the school curriculum. It requires healthier communities. Violence against others thrives in the absence of democracy, respect for human rights and good governance. Violence against self thrives in the absence of self-respect, a sense of belonging and hope.

Most suicide attempts are "unsuccessful"—a problematic term. They are a cry for help. And they are usually preceded by other cries for help that, all too often, go unheeded. More often than not, suicide has its roots in mental illness and in other social ills such as loneliness and hopelessness. Yet mental-health services are grossly underfunded, particularly services for children and adolescents, where intervention can have the greatest impact. There was talk, in the wake of the Dawson shootings, of equipping schools with metal detectors and armed guards. However, the money would be far better spent on getting nurses, psychologists and counsellors into schools, where they can do prevention work. Yet we don't have these discussions. Why? Because talking about mental-health issues makes us terribly uncomfortable, and suicide doubly so.

A murderer can easily be classified as evil, a criminal. But what to make of someone who turns the violence inward? Are they evil, too? Are they criminal? No, overwhelmingly, people who are considering suicide are sick and in need of care. Suicide is a health problem just like infectious diseases such as SARS and chronic illnesses such as heart disease. Like them, suicide should be the subject of health research and media stories. Yet suicides warrant virtually no media coverage— either individually or collectively. In fact, most news outlets have policies (official and unofficial) to not cover suicides lest they provoke copycat deaths.

Little evidence exists that stories of suicide provoke more suicides.

Or that news coverage of murders sparks more murders, for that matter. But a double standard remains. The homicide at Dawson College generated unprecedented levels of Canadian media coverage because it was unusual—very public and involving several guns. Two young people died tragically that day: an eighteen-year-old woman was savagely slain, and a twenty-five-year-old man culminated a violent outburst by taking his own life. All the sympathy, the tears and the concern have been for De Sousa. But, from a public-health perspective, just as much—if not more—attention should be paid to the suicide of Kimveer Gill.

Fewer than two homicides a day occur in Canada, but there are more than ten suicides daily—each of them a violent act, and each of them a failure of the public-health system.

Burying the story won't stop suicide

One Saturday morning—it could be any weekend because it's all too common—a nineteen-year-old student jumped to his death from the fifteenth floor of a residence building at the University of Ottawa. Is that news? If so, how detailed should the news reports be? Will drawing attention to the tragedy be helpful or harmful? How to cover suicides poses one of the most difficult ethical dilemmas for journalists and editors.

There were 3,926 suicides in Canada in 2012, the most recent year for which detailed data are available. What a tragic waste of life. Should we be turning a blind eye to this carnage so as to not offend sensibilities? Or should we be shining a light on suicide deaths—most of them preventable—to highlight the underlying cause, which is often untreated mental illness?

The Canadian Psychiatric Association has published guidelines for media reporting on suicide. The guidelines have, as their premise, a statement that "media coverage of suicide is proven to lead to copycat suicides." The evidence suggests that media stories about suicide can be harmful, particularly if they are given prominent play in the newspaper or on a newscast, if the stories are repeated often and if they involve a celebrity. One study, for example, showed an increase in suicides following the suicide of Gaétan Girouard, a high-profile Quebec TV personality, and the reverential coverage that followed.

In its media guidelines, the psychiatrists' group urges reporters and editors to avoid the following: giving details of the suicide method; using the word *suicide* in the headline; publishing photos or "admiration of the deceased"; repetitive, excessive or front-page coverage; "exciting" reporting; citing romanticized or simplistic reasons for the suicide; suggesting that suicide is unexplainable; and approval of the suicide. The position paper essentially calls on journalists to sweep uncomfortable details under the carpet, to dehumanize the dead. It is also not realistic, especially when high-profile figures like Kurt Cobain and Robin Williams are dying by suicide.

In response, a group of journalists produced their own guidelines. Not surprisingly, the approach is markedly different from that of psychiatrists. In a document titled *Mindset: Reporting on Mental Health*, they argue that the longstanding taboo about reporting on suicide is outdated and is harmful because it perpetuates stigma. Journalists, they argue, "should cover suicides the way they cover murders, seeking to find answers about the causes, while mourning the dead, flaws and all." In other words, cover suicide like every other health and social issue. They also take the position that the evidence on copycat suicides is epidemiologically weak, and that reporting tends to influence the *method* of suicide more than it prompts more suicides. The *Mindset* guide urges reporters to watch their language, in particular to avoid prejudicial phrases like "committed suicide" (an expression that harkens back to the days when suicide was a crime and a sin) and, instead of euphemistic phrases like "died suddenly," use precise language like "took her own life."

Regardless of their philosophical differences, psychiatrists and journalists agree on a number of key issues, notably that there is rarely any need to go into the details about the methods used, and that news stories should avoid romanticizing the act or speculating on why people kill themselves because the reasons are often complex and/or not clear. They agree too that a tremendous opportunity exists to educate the public about mental-health problems and their treatment. When articles are published about suicide they should, ideally, feature information on how to get help if a person is suicidal and remind readers that suicide is usually the result of treatable mental illness.

So how did the media fare in covering the University of Ottawa death? The *Ottawa Citizen* published an article titled "Students seek answers in on-campus death." It did not name the student or even use the word *suicide*, stating that he "fell to his death." CBC Ottawa published a story on its website titled "U of O students mourn suicide victim." It revealed the student's name and spoke to his friends, who spoke of him with admiration. The broadcaster also published a photo of a memorial featuring an emotional goodbye card. The *Fulcrum*, U of O's student newspaper, published only a small article titled "University reacts to campus tragedy." The paper published the student's name but it did not use the word *suicide*. Most of its article focused on the availability of counselling and mental-health services on campus.

Emma Godmere, then-editor of the *Fulcrum*, noted that within minutes of the student's suicide, she received the news electronically. "I got a text, a BlackBerry message and an e-mail right away," she said. Later, there were Facebook posts and tweets (some rumoured to have featured pictures of the corpse). This is a reminder that, no matter how well-intentioned, the Canadian Psychiatric Association's guidelines are a bit anachronistic in the age of social media.

Let's face it—with technological advances and shifting mores, privacy is not what it used to be. Neither is suicide. The article in the *Fulcrum* did not trigger copycat suicides; nor did the Facebook posts and other cyberspace exchanges or the memorial. But they did raise awareness. Maybe the taboos are finally being shattered. Maybe by talking more openly about mental illness we can prevent suicides. Burying our heads in the sand and self-censoring our stories certainly has not worked.

Suicide should not be an occupational hazard for doctors

On November 17, 2014, the inanimate body of Émilie Marchand was found in a parked car in the north end of Montreal. The twenty-seven-year-old medical resident at the University of Montreal died by suicide from an overdose of the painkiller hydromorphone. Unlike most suicides, Marchand's death garnered a lot of media attention. It occurred at a time when the dysfunctional administration at U of M–affiliated hospitals was under scrutiny, and came on the heels of a damning report by the university's ombudsman about another medical student's suicide.

One year later, Quebec coroner Jean Brochu weighed in, pointing a finger at the University of Montreal for sitting idly by while a sick, troubled student was "slipping slowly and solitarily toward a dead-end of desperation." While his report looked at a specific case, the coroner noted that it was part of a much larger problem—astronomical rates of depression among medical students and residents, coupled with the troubling reality that as many as one in seven had seriously contemplated suicide.

Suicide is now considered an occupational hazard for physicians: about four hundred doctors take their own lives in the United States annually, as do a few dozen in Canada. And the problems begin early: medical students face significantly higher rates of burnout, depression and mental illness than those in the general population. Medical students—and residents in particular—face tremendous pressure, including punishing exams, a cutthroat atmosphere and gruelling hours.

Stress is not the sole explanation. As both the coroner and the ombudsman noted in their reports, the medical classroom and workplace are brutal: bullying and psychological harassment are commonplace in schools and hospitals, and the stigma about mental illness is pervasive in the medical profession. Medical education is too often imbued with a macho attitude that learners have to be broken down and toughened up and that those who can't take it are weak and unworthy.

Perversely, many physicians take pride in this boot-camp mentality. When efforts were made to eliminate the insane hundred-hour workweeks of residents, old-timers quietly (and sometimes not so quietly) dismissed the younger generation as wimps. Even Quebec health minister Dr. Gaétan Barrette, when asked about medical-school suicides, reacted dismissively, saying, "The pressure they are dealing with is a lot less than it was fifteen years ago." In fact, what's different today is not that young people are weaker, it is that expectations are much higher and isolation is much greater, in spite of (or perhaps because of) so-called social media. Medical students and residents are also headed into a world of uncertainty, not one where they are guaranteed a life of privilege. At least now there is open recognition and discussion of the problem, whereas in the past, when residents and doctors killed themselves, it was hushed up. But while the system has become adept at collecting data on depression and suicide, it has done little that is concrete to offer help and invest in prevention.

Émilie Marchand, like all her classmates, had stellar marks and, from the time she was in high school, had dedicated herself heart and soul to the goal of becoming a doctor—in her case a specialist in internal medicine. When she was in medical school she was diagnosed with a personality disorder and, in residency, suffered from bouts of depression so severe that she had to be hospitalized. She also had made a previous suicide attempt, using the same drug, hydromorphone. But Marchand continued her studies full bore and—her friends testified later—lived in mortal fear that her illness would be exposed and her career derailed.

Increasingly, research is showing that so-called super-performers, like those attracted to medical school, are particularly vulnerable. Paradoxically, the very qualities that make someone a good doctor— empathy, caring and perfectionism—make them vulnerable to burnout, depression and suicide.

The students attracted to medical school are among the best and brightest of their generation. They are smart, talented and driven.

But many are also anxious, overwhelmed and lost—sick, not weak. We cannot simply respond to the wounded healers with the age-old admonishment, *medice, cura te ipsum* (physician, heal thyself). We must create an environment where our future doctors can learn to heal, beginning with caring for themselves.

----∿----

The "freedom" to be sick and the right to be well

C an we, in a democratic society, justify incarcerating people who have committed no crime? Is forcing sick people to take medication against their will legal, and constitutional? The answer to those questions is yes, according to a 2016 ruling by the Court of Appeal of Ontario, which rejected a legal challenge to what is commonly known as Brian's Law. The court upheld provisions of the Ontario Mental Health Act, which allows for people suffering from severe mental illness to be committed to psychiatric institutions for treatment, and the Health Care Consent Act, which allows for community treatment orders (CTOs) that mandate continuing treatment, usually involving medication. The decision—which is being appealed to the Supreme Court—has potentially far-reaching ramifications because most jurisdictions have some form of committal on their books, and five provinces use CTOs.

A little background is needed to situate the debate. In 1995, Ottawa sportscaster Brian Smith was shot to death by Jeffrey Arenburg, an untreated schizophrenia sufferer who heard voices and felt that killing a broadcaster would silence them. An inquest concluded that Arenburg should have been in hospital, but the law was too weak. In 2000, Ontario adopted the new Brian's Law, which beefed up the law.

The Empowerment Council Systemic Advocates in Addictions and Mental Health, a group of self-described "psychiatric survivors," challenged the law. The applicant in the case was Karlene Thompson, a fifty-nine-year-old former teacher who was diagnosed with schizophrenia in 1973 and was hospitalized at least thirteen times up to 2000. She was hospitalized again after she was found living in a squalid rooming house where she collected her feces and urine in plastic bags. Thompson was released on a CTO that obliged her to take antipsychotic drugs. She did until 2003, after which she became delusional and deteriorated physically. Then the legal battle began. (Thompson eventually moved back to her native Jamaica to avoid treatment, but the case proceeded.)

Such cases are complex, but in essence, the key issue was the purpose of the legislation: is it intended to bolster public safety or to improve the treatment of patients who are seriously mentally ill? In upholding a ruling by Justice Edward Belobaba of the Ontario Supreme Court, the appeals court agreed that the law is clearly designed to help people and not punish them.

Parents and caregivers of people with severe mental illness have long been frustrated by civil libertarians who argue that individual rights—including the right to refuse treatment—are paramount. That's because those with severe mental illness often have a symptom called anosognosia—a lack of awareness that they are actually sick. Treatment is "forced" on them because they don't have the capacity to make a rational decision. That is not cruel and unusual punishment. On the contrary, it is humane and compassionate. Involuntary committal to a psychiatric institution is a last resort; it is also a rarity, usually reserved for those who commit serious acts of violence and are judged not criminally responsible. For the most part, people with severe mental illness who refuse treatment and who become a risk to themselves or others as a result end up with CTOs. And it should be noted that physicians or family members cannot impose these conditions on a whim; an elaborate legal process needs to be followed, with appeal processes up to and including the Consent and Capacity Board.

Between 2000 and 2010 in Ontario, the number of CTOs issued annually ranged from 656 to 1,093. The mandatory treatment lasts, on average, 1.9 years. But most CTOs are renewed because those affected tend to be the sickest of the sick. Community treatment orders are far from perfect, and this has been well documented. But, if anything, they are underused. Too many sick people are still caught in a revolving door between treatment and illness. We resist because the notion of treating people against their will (even if they are irrational) sticks in our craw. Currently, about five thousand people in Ontario are under mandatory treatment, most of them living in the community.

In addition, drugs used to treat those with severe mental illness, especially antipsychotics, are far from perfect. They can cause massive weight gain and increase the risk of diabetes and heart disease. But again, it's a balancing of risks. Harming the heart is an unfortunate but fair trade-off if it prevents a person from wallowing daily in his own feces, harming others or killing himself. And the imperfection of drugs does not invalidate the law or undermine its purpose.

Without proper treatment, people with severe mental illness live dismal lives, usually on the streets or in prison. They die deaths by a thousand cuts, deaths by a thousand pills, deaths by a thousand missed opportunities for care. The most urgent question people have when their loved ones are in the clutches of a devastating illness like schizophrenia is, "How do I get them help?" CTOs are a necessary tool when the situation becomes desperate.

Of course, when the state behaves in a coercive fashion against an individual, we should be concerned, and doubly so when that power is enshrined in legislation. But the interventions allowed under Brian's Law are justified and necessary; they meet the test of reasonable limits to the freedoms guaranteed in the Charter of Rights and Freedoms. But those are technical legal matters. The Ontario court ruling is important, above all, because it reminds us that individual autonomy needs to be balanced against the right to be well. The "freedom" to be sick is a false freedom.

Canada's ugly mental-health secret

I magine that you have a child or teenager who is suicidal, suffering from depression, severe anxiety, an eating disorder, a drug addiction or another mental-health problem. You can seek the care of a psychiatrist, a service covered by medicare, but the wait for an appointment is months, maybe even a year. Or you can seek the help of a psychologist or social worker who also does therapy. There is no wait but services are not covered by medicare, so you must pay out-of-pocket, roughly $130 an hour. That is the unenviable choice Canadian parents face every day. What do you do?

The well-to-do pay. The middle-class scrape together the money the best they can, sacrificing so their child can get care. And those without the means wait, or do without care. "What we have today in Canada is a two-tier mental-health system in which kids are the victim," says Michael Kirby, the founding chairman of Partners for Mental Health. "This is a situation that offends my values as a Canadian." What troubles him even more is the breadth of the problem. An estimated 1.2 million Canadian children are affected by mental illness. Yet only one in four gets appropriate treatment. Access to care, speedy or otherwise, is not the only issue. Stigma, denial and fear play a part, too.

Kirby, a former Canadian senator and tireless advocate for better mental-health care, planned to do something about it. He pieced together a plan, and he knocked on the doors of federal, provincial and territorial health ministers to get them on board. The idea was straightforward: get governments to commit to pay for psychological counselling for children and youth for up to eight sessions—eight being the number most employee-assistance programs and private insurance plans will pay for. That would be roughly $1,000 per child, or up to $500 million if everyone who could theoretically benefit from treatment took up the offer. That may have seemed like a pipe dream at a time when governments were trying to hold the line on health spending.

But Kirby had an impressive track record. For example, the principal recommendation of the landmark report produced by his Senate committee in 2007, *Out of the Shadows at Last*, was the creation of a mental-health commission. The federal government heeded that request, and $150 million followed. The bold At Home/Chez Soi research project, which examined how to tackle the pervasive problems of homelessness and mental illness and addiction among the homeless, received an additional $110 million in funding.

Kirby's principal argument in promoting the expansion of treatment of mental illness in young people was that the investment would pay off in spades. "Almost all mental-health problems begin in the young, before the age of twenty-four," he noted. "If you get them early, you avoid a lifetime of problems and costs." That is language governments understand. It is especially true because of the growing recognition that mental-health problems, beyond being a personal burden, are a blow to productivity and a drain on the economy. In fact, it has been estimated that mental illness costs the economy more than $50 billion a year. One of the reasons that number is so high is precisely because problems are so pervasive—an estimated 6.7 million Canadians suffer from mental illness at any given time—and illness tends to hit people hardest in their prime work years. Nipping problems in the bud should be appealing to cost-conscious governments.

After stepping down from the Mental Health Commission of Canada, Kirby turned his attention to creating Partners for Mental Health, which he envisages as a social movement that will one day do for mental health what the Canadian Cancer Society has done for cancer and the Heart and Stroke Foundation has done for cardiovascular disease. In addition to tackling the problem of two-tier access to mental-health services, Partners for Mental Health is beating the drum for a national youth suicide prevention fund. And in 2012, Parliament passed Bill C-300, the Federal Framework for Suicide Prevention Act. It essentially called on Ottawa to develop a plan to combat suicide, but did not include a commitment of money, and the result is that Canada still has no suicide prevention strategy.

About thirty-nine hundred Canadians die by suicide each year, including almost six hundred young people. In 2016, Partners for Mental Health called on governments to invest $100 million over four years in suicide prevention, most of it for education programs and crisis intervention. In both cases, Kirby called for provinces and territories to take the lead and for Ottawa to offer dollar-for-dollar matching funds. That was a good strategic move from a wily political veteran who knows Ottawa is reluctant to create programs, and provinces are hesitant to act without federal dollars. So far, there has been no firm commitment to funding either psychological care or suicide prevention, but action seems imminent, as new money for mental health has become the central negotiating point in talks about a new Health Accord.

"Governments have invested in me and my ideas big-time and I'm grateful for that," Kirby said. "But I would like them to invest a little more—this time in young people, in the future. This is my last kick at the can, telling governments that they can do right by kids, they can create a better future."

Robin Williams gives a voice to a silent killer

The media world changed dramatically in the twenty years between the suicides of Kurt Cobain and Robin Williams, but there is no question the coverage of mental-health issues, and suicide in particular, is infinitely better. When Kurt Cobain died of a self-inflicted shotgun blast to the head in April 1994, he was dubbed a "casualty of success." The Nirvana singer was described, alternately, as a rock star who died living on the edge and as a charter member of "the stupid club," the infamous series of musicians who died at twenty-seven, at the height of their success. Snide references were made to Cobain's drug use and abuse, but little was mentioned of the severe depression he suffered and of his struggles with addiction. In fact, most media reported that he used heroin to treat "chronic stomach pain."

Contrast that with the reporting on the death of Robin Williams, who died by asphyxiation due to hanging in August of 2014. Much of the reporting—even in the early hours after the news broke—focused on the actor's diagnosis of bipolar disorder, his history of depression and how he self-medicated with alcohol and drugs such as cocaine. Aside from some predictable gibberish from trolls, there was little talk of weakness and ungratefulness for success. Rather, the emphasis was on how depression can afflict anyone, even the rich, the famous and the funny. Social media such as Facebook and Twitter overflowed not only with tributes to Williams, but with links to resources for those suffering from depression and suicidal thoughts.

By this time, in-depth articles were already being published about the underfunding of mental-health research, the long waits for care, and how some specific demographic groups were at much greater risk of suicide—in particular, men of Williams's age, in their sixties. (Men are four times as likely to die by suicide as women, largely because of their reluctance to seek treatment.) The breadth and the sophistication of the media coverage has been heartwarming. You can virtually feel the knowledge of depression growing and the stigma surrounding mental illness evaporating, and that may well be Williams's most lasting legacy. But the suicide of a well-known public figure, combined with the ubiquity of social media, poses some real ethical challenges, chief among them, how much information is enough—or too much?

For a long time, the media either did not cover suicide or wrote about self-inflicted deaths euphemistically—for example, "died suddenly." This was due to a strange mix of puritanism, respect and shame. Many of those self-imposed barriers crumbled with Cobain's death—one of the first celebrity deaths of the social-media age. Loved ones of those who died by suicide (especially parents of teens) also challenged media silence because they viewed it as a barrier to others getting help. Journalists also operated under the belief that writing about suicide would lead to more suicide, the so-called contagion effect. But in recent years, editors and reporters have pulled their heads out of the sand and decided to focus on reporting factually and respectfully on suicide. Groups such as Associated Press editors and the Canadian Journalism Forum on Violence and Trauma have developed their own guidelines.

This guidance is necessary because we live in what is essentially the post-privacy age, as demonstrated by Marin County Sheriff Lieutenant Keith Boyd, who described Williams's death in painful detail at a live broadcast press conference. (Police also released gruesome photos after Cobain's death.) The challenge for the media is not to linger on those details, but rather to use them as a springboard to discuss the underlying causes of suicide and the improvements that are needed in prevention and treatment.

About 41,500 Americans (and another 3,900 Canadians) die by suicide annually, making it one of the leading causes of death. About 90 percent of people who die by suicide are suffering from untreated or undertreated mental illness. (Williams was suffering from severe depression, as well as Lewy body disease, a form of dementia. His autopsy showed that he had two drugs in his system, the antidepressant Mirtazapine and the antipsychotic Seroquel.)

In recent years, the "tears of a clown" metaphor has sometimes been used to underscore how sufferers of depression, like Williams, often wear an outward mask of joy to hide their inner pain. As a society, we have also been hiding behind a mask, failing to acknowledge that mental illness—and untreated mental illness in particular—is a public-health crisis that rivals physical diseases like cancer and heart disease. Suicide is, by and large, a silent killer. It was given a voice—at least temporarily—by the man of many voices, Robin Williams. Are we listening?

Eating disorders: A scourge in need of a strategy

Eating disorders are the single most deadly mental illness: between 10 and 15 percent of young women hospitalized for treatment of anorexia or bulimia will be dead within ten years. Somewhere between 600,000 and 990,000 Canadians suffer from eating disorders. Yet they remain among the most neglected and misunderstood of all health conditions. Those were just two of the shocking findings of the parliamentary Standing Committee on the Status of Women. The committee's November 2014 seventy-five-page report, *Eating Disorders Among Girls and Women in Canada*, was much anticipated by parents and clinicians alike, who know all too well the direness of the situation.

Imagine that your teenaged daughter is starving to death—literally, not figuratively—but the wait for treatment is more than a year. Or imagine that your child is suicidal but deemed "not sick enough" for hospital admission because of a shortage of beds. The number of girls between ten and nineteen hospitalized for treatment of eating disorders soared by 42 percent between 2012 and 2014, but the system still can't keep up. Shortages are widespread and chronic. "There is something inherently wrong with a public health-care system that often only becomes available when someone is on death's door," Elaine Stevenson told the committee. At age twenty-four, her daughter Alyssa died of anorexia, like about fifteen hundred other young Canadian women each year.

The protracted wait times are doubly perverse because it's well established that early intervention—counselling for girls (and boys) who have disordered eating, rather than full-blown eating disorders—can be a very effective prevention tool. The frustration continues once patients are admitted for treatment. The first order of business is refeeding—getting patients with eating disorders to eat three square meals a day rather than, for example, binging and purging. But the feeding needs to be accompanied with psychiatric or psychological therapy to address the underlying mental-health problem, and few hospitals have the resources to offer that care. Of the forty-one hundred psychiatrists practising in Canada, only twelve specialize in the treatment of eating disorders.

The most effective treatment is a combination of cognitive behavioural therapy (CBT) and family-based therapy (FBT), supplemented with nutritional counselling. Eating tends to be a family-based activity, which is why the involvement of parents and siblings is essential to recovery. But CBT and FBT are not covered by medicare. Therapy costs anywhere from $80 to $250 an hour. Consider that several hours of therapy a week can be necessary and that treatment for these stubborn conditions routinely lasts two to seven years. Even then, only about half of sufferers fully recover.

While hospital resources are scarce, community-based help for people with eating disorders is virtually non-existent. Consumer groups like the National Initiative for Eating Disorders survive on a wing and a prayer, driven by personal suffering. Dr. Blake Woodside, medical director of the eating-disorder program at Toronto General Hospital, told the committee that the cause of all this is "egregious discrimination" against a demographic group with no political clout. "If there were waits like this of four to six months for prostate cancer treatment, there would be a national outcry. There would be marches in the streets," he said. But because eating disorders affect teenaged girls, there is no outrage or political action.

Those called to speak before the committee all had, more or less, the same message: a pan-Canadian strategy is needed to tackle this growing scourge. That includes better prevention, education, treatment and follow-up care. Many stated that the starting point should be a national registry, to get a better sense of who is (and isn't) getting care, and a robust research program to help develop better treatment and support. What the committee provided, however, was twenty-five spineless recommendations urging the federal government to "consider," "encourage" and "recognize" a number of self-evident needs. Those are do-nothing weasel words—another example of the then-Conservative government's obsessive desire to not involve itself in health care regardless of the harm its neglect caused patients. Both the New Democrats and Liberals wrote dissenting opinions and tried to publicize the report the government wanted buried.

Young women (and men) with eating disorders don't need indifference and platitudes—they need concrete changes to the health system to, in the words of dissenting Liberal committee member Kirsty Duncan, "steer them through the confusing and overwhelming world in which they are embroiled."

—⌒⌒—

The torture of solitary segregation has no place in a society that respects human rights

S olitary confinement can, for short periods, be an acceptable form of punishment. But the consensus, nationally and internationally, is that *prolonged segregation*—the Canadian term for locking away a prisoner alone for twenty-two or twenty-three hours a day—cannot be considered anything but cruel and unusual punishment, particularly for young people and those suffering from mental illness or suicidal thoughts. Yet in Canada, the practice is still commonplace, and it was heartily defended by the "law and order" Conservative government under Stephen Harper.

There are over fifteen thousand inmates in federal prisons, about 850 of whom are in segregation at any given time. Each year, 46 percent of female prisoners and 26 percent of male prisoners spend at least one day in either "disciplinary segregation" (punishment for some transgression of prison rules) or "administrative segregation" (because they are considered a risk to themselves or others, which is generally a euphemism for saying a prisoner is suicidal or severely mentally ill). Data from provincial and territorial jails is almost impossible to come by, although a lawsuit revealed that, in two Ontario jails alone, sixteen hundred prisoners had spent time in solitary over a five-month period. Most troubling of all is that young offenders are twice as likely to find themselves in solitary as adult prisoners. And there is every indication that those sent to segregation most often and for the longest periods are precisely those who will suffer the most harm.

In late 2014, *The Globe and Mail* highlighted the heart-rending case of Eddie Snowshoe, a mentally ill indigenous man who spent 162 days straight in segregation before taking his own life. His case recalls the tragic death of Ashley Smith, a young woman who spent, mind-bogglingly, over one thousand days alone in a cell before killing herself as guards watched on a video monitor and refused to intervene, no less. (The United Nations says that anything more than fifteen consecutive days of solitary confinement should be considered torture. In Canada, the average stay is twenty-seven days.) Aside from drawing attention to the vulgar inhumanity of prolonged segregation, these cases are a reminder that our prisons have become, to a disturbing extent, de facto psychiatric institutions.

While psych hospitals have isolation rooms, they are used sparingly and as a respite for those suffering from active psychosis and in danger of harming themselves. Prolonged isolation is no longer used in medical settings because the evidence of the physical and psychological harm it can cause is overwhelming, from weakening the immune system to triggering psychosis. As counterintuitive as it may seem, isolation is far more likely to cause aggressive behaviour than curtail it. So why is the practice used—and used more frequently—despite these facts?

Solitary confinement has a long and fascinating history. The idea was conceived by the Quakers—a sociable, peace-loving group—in the late 1700s as a humane alternative to the popular practices of chain gangs, stockades and public hangings. They believed solitude would afford an ideal opportunity to seek forgiveness from God—that it would bring penitence (hence the term *penitentiary*). But it became obvious early on that isolation did a lot more damage to the brain than it did good to the soul.

Segregation has been harmful and ineffective for more than two centuries, yet it seems that Correctional Service Canada didn't get the memo. Section 718 of the Criminal Code lays out pretty clearly the fundamental purpose for sending an offender to prison:

(a) to denounce unlawful conduct;
(b) to deter the offender and other persons from committing offences;
(c) to separate offenders from society, where necessary;
(d) to assist in rehabilitating offenders;
(e) to provide reparations for harm done to victims or to the community; and
(f) to promote a sense of responsibility in offenders, and acknowledgement of the harm done to victims and to the community.

Beyond those sensible goals, it basically comes down to one's philosophical view of the primary purpose of incarceration: should it be punitive or rehabilitative? Most prisoners will be released back into society, so it makes sense—ethically, economically and practically—to rehabilitate. Still, the Hammurabian approach of an eye for an eye, with a side order of vengeful retribution, still holds some sway. The remaining question, then, is, how much punishment is enough? Imprisonment is essentially a denial of freedom for a set period of time, reflective of the severity of a crime. But if you want a prisoner to reintegrate into society, that denial cannot be absolute. Prolonged segregation is designed to humiliate and dehumanize, not rehabilitate.

Presumably, we've moved beyond the era when prisons were Dickensian warehouses of torture. And segregation is torture, particularly when inflicted on children and the mentally ill. It is not an acceptable practice in a country that purports to respect human rights.

If we send soldiers to war, we owe them peace of mind

War changes men and women. It leaves wounds—physical and mental. We have developed countless weapons to kill and maim and, as a counterpoint, sophisticated body armour to minimize injuries and amazing medical treatments to piece wounded warriors together again. But while we can prevent and treat many visible physical injuries, what about the oft-invisible mental harms? Where is the bulletproof vest for the mind? How do you heal the minds of soldiers haunted by what they have seen and felt?

As long as there has been war, there has been lasting psychological harm and, tragically, despair and suicide among veterans. The language we use now—post-traumatic stress disorder instead of shell shock, and depression instead of malingering—is more precise. What is taking longer to change is the stigma—the whispered suggestions that PTSD afflicts the weak—and reluctance among tough guys (and gals) to seek help.

Today we do a somewhat better job of body counts. One hundred and fifty-eight soldiers died during Canada's mission to the Afghanistan war; at least seventy-one more took their own lives, eight in the theatre of war and the balance when they returned home. The former have been treated as heroes, the latter as less worthy of mourning and commemoration—a hurtful double standard. Soldiers suffering from post-traumatic stress disorder often face dismissive, penny-pinching treatment when they reach out for care, and their families fare even worse. In contrast to the combat deaths, the suicide deaths have been hushed up, compounding the pain. That discriminatory response needs to be corrected. But in addition to helping soldiers and veterans currently suffering from PTSD, much larger questions need to be addressed: can we prevent PTSD or, at the very least, minimize its impacts?

Post-traumatic stress disorder is an anxiety disorder that some people acquire after witnessing a traumatic event. In recent years, much research has been conducted on and much has been learned about PTSD, in large part due to the massive deployment of US troops in Iraq and Afghanistan and the retrospective analysis of the experiences of Vietnam War veterans. "Fight or flight" is a healthy reaction to danger and usually serves us well. But people with PTSD remain stressed or frightened even when they are no longer in danger, a process called "fear conditioning." While most people will suffer at least one traumatic event in their lifetime, most do not suffer long-term effects. Humans tend to be resilient. But a significant minority will suffer from chronic, unremitting stress and anxiety. In the words of Afghanistan veteran Russ Lee, who struggles with PTSD, "When the combat mission is over, the war is fought inside of us."

Almost one in five Vietnam War veterans suffered from PTSD. Researchers found three factors that predisposed soldiers to the illness:

· severity of exposure—the more horrific the things soldiers witnessed, the greater the risk;
· history of childhood abuse—soldiers who were physically or sexually assaulted, meaning they had already suffered trauma; and
· history of substance abuse in the family, another form of trauma.

Other research hints that some people's brains are anatomically better able to recover from trauma. Understanding the roots of resilience suggests that screening could reveal which soldiers are predisposed to PTSD—not with the goal of excluding them, but of ensuring they are monitored and get follow-up care.

The US Armed Forces have tried a number of methods to prevent PTSD, but most have proven ineffective, according to a report from the Institute of Medicine. The clear message that emerges from research is that swift response to trauma is important. PTSD symptoms usually arise within three months and, if untreated, tend to grow worse with time. The US National Center for Biotechnology Information, in a comprehensive analysis of PTSD treatments, found that drugs are largely ineffective, except to treat specific symptoms. What work best are psychological interventions such as cognitive behavioural therapy (CBT), cognitive processing therapy (CPT) and prolonged exposure (PE), all of which help patients understand the impact of trauma and restructure their beliefs. While these approaches are effective, they take time (about a dozen sessions for most) and money (psychological care is not generally covered under medicare).

Those with the most severe forms of PTSD also suffer from persistent suicidal thoughts, which can require institutional care. The suicide rate among military personnel is more than twice that of the general population, and PTSD can be a precipitating factor. In exchange for their service, members of the military should be provided with the care they need. Not care that is cursory, but the care that is necessary for their recovery. That is the social contract the Canadian Armed Forces, and by extension, the federal government, have been failing to honour.

If we are going to spend on war, we also need to invest in peace of mind. Thanks to a few brave veterans and advocates, the invisible disability of PTSD (and the related tragedy of suicide) is now visible. What remains is for Canada to cast off its wilful blindness.

CHAPTER 3

Drugs

Drugs aren't commodities to be
hustled like cars and cookies

One of the most important and overlooked recommendations of the US advisory committee that, in 2005, held public hearings on the safety of Vioxx and other COX-2 inhibitors was a call to ban all advertising of the popular painkillers. The panel members made it clear that advertising played a central role in this debacle.

Vioxx and Celebrex were among the most heavily advertised drugs in history. Their main claim to fame, touted in slick ads, was that they were safer than cheaper painkillers such as ibuprofen when, in reality, they increased the risk of heart attack and stroke. Advertising, in no small measure, led to the gross overprescription of these drugs to people with arthritis and other painful conditions. And it was telling that, when questions began to be raised about the safety of Vioxx, its maker, Merck & Co., responded by bolstering the ad campaign for the drug, not by commissioning research to investigate scientists' concerns. Vioxx was more heavily advertised than Pepsi and Budweiser, and that is a perversity.

The advisory panel served up an important reminder that advertising prescription drugs is a privilege, a lucrative privilege that, in the name of public safety, can be denied. Currently, only two countries allow direct-to-consumer advertising of prescription drugs, the United States and New Zealand.

The Canadian Food and Drugs Act explicitly prohibits such advertising—sort of. In 1999, however, Health Canada "reinterpreted" the act and related regulations and concluded, in the words of then–health minister Allan Rock, that "two types of prescription-drug ads may be disseminated to the consumers under the existing regulatory provisions: 1) reminder ads—where the name of a prescription drug is mentioned, but no reference to a disease state appears in the ad; or 2) help-seeking ads—where a disease state is discussed, but no reference is made to a specific prescription-drug product."

That is why ads like those featuring an unseen couple frolicking on the sofa with popcorn overflowing on the stovetop, followed by the single word, Pfizer, have become ubiquitous. (They make a little blue pill called Viagra.) It is why, in the pages of newspapers, you can see ads that depict the corpse of a middle-aged woman who is not obese with a toe tag showing her cause of death as "heart attack" and urging consumers to "ask your doctor"—not-too-subtle advertising for the cholesterol-lowering medication Lipitor. The rules are such that "reminder" and "help-seeking" ads are permitted.

Critics of Canada's law argue that it is hopelessly outdated, that consumers would be better served by advertising that encourages dialogue between patients and physicians and provides accessible health information. Meanwhile, opponents of direct-to-consumer advertising argue that no evidence exists that advertising prescription drugs has ever resulted in better health care or more responsible decision-making by consumers. But there is plenty of evidence showing a direct and disturbing correlation between promotion and prescription—and unnecessary prescription in particular.

In 2016, we spent $31 billion on prescriptions. Advertising can be a powerful influence. The makers of Claritin, an allergy pill, found that for every ad dollar spent, their sales increased by $3.50. But widespread direct-to-consumer advertising increases the cost to individuals, to employee insurance plans and to government drug plans. Without much doubt, it also increases adverse events related to drugs. According to the *Canadian Medical Association Journal*, prescription drug sales would soar in Canada if us-style advertising were allowed; that's because when patients specifically request a drug, they are seventeen times more likely to be prescribed that drug.

The only real beneficiaries of advertising are pharmaceutical companies and the media. The *CMAJ* (which is allowed to run drug ads because its primary readership is physicians and not the general public) estimates that mainstream media would rake in at least $360 million in revenues annually from prescription drug ads. The public—and the public-health system—does not benefit from prescription drug advertising in the mainstream media. On the contrary, the evidence suggests it is bad for their health. That is why the regulator, Health Canada, should drop the notion of relaxing restrictions and turn its attention to enforcing the laws that currently exist, even extending them to non-prescription drugs and supplements (where all manner of quackery is currently tolerated), and to advertising to physicians (an area rife with conflicts of interest). One of Health Canada's key responsibilities is to ensure that the drugs on the Canadian market are safe. That must include ensuring that the prescription-drug information conveyed to consumers is accurate and balanced.

Among other things, the Vioxx saga reminded us that drugs are not just another commodity to be flogged like cars and cookies. Vioxx contributed to the death of as many as sixty-one thousand Americans (and another four thousand to seven thousand Canadians) during the five years it was on the market—and those numbers were made worse by massive marketing campaigns. Consumers want good, no-nonsense information about drugs, but the last place they are going to get that is from an orgy of drug advertising.

Drop that prescription pad

Primum non nocere. That Latin maxim, roughly translated as "above all, do no harm," is a key element of the Hippocratic Oath. One of the foundational elements of medical ethics is non-maleficence, the notion that when treating a patient, it may be preferable to *not* do something, or even do nothing at all, if the intervention risks causing more harm than good. Yet in our modern era, with its dizzying technological innovations, ready access to a cornucopia of drugs and impatience driven by the jolts-per-minute pace of daily life, the guiding maxim has become "Do something. Do anything."

You see it every day in medical practice. No one wants to leave a physician's office without a prescription or a high-tech test. Everybody wants to be screened so they can nip cancer in the bud or catch Alzheimer's early, even when this information can do more harm than good. The Nike "Just do it" catch phrase and the consumerist philosophy that more is always better may carry the day on TV dramas such as *House*, but it has no place in real-life medicine. Acting swiftly and firmly may provide succour, at least temporarily, but every action has an equal and often greater reaction.

We seem—in medicine as in life—to have lost the precious ability to ponder. To wait. To utter the three magic words, "I don't know." To wisely do nothing until we know more, or until nature takes its course. The result is an epidemic of overtreatment that is both financially costly and physically harmful. The reality was exposed in a sobering book by journalist Shannon Brownlee titled *Overtreated: Why Too Much Medicine Is Making Us Sicker and Poorer* (Bloomsbury, 2010). Her work was prescient. In May 2011, the Good Stewardship Working Group—physicians who believe good care can be delivered cost-effectively—published a list of commonly used tests and treatments that are unnecessary. Then, in November 2011, a group of academics costed out the savings that would come from eliminating a dozen wasteful interventions—a whopping $6.8 billion a year in the United States—and published their results in the Archives of Internal Medicine. Choosing Wisely, an initiative of the American Board of Internal Medicine Foundation, then took up the cause. It asked medical specialty societies to identify five overused tests or treatments and so far have generated four hundred recommendations. Anecdotally, Choosing Wisely is changing practice and saving money, at least within individual institutions that have embraced the approach. But it's too soon to tell whether a fundamental cultural shift has occurred.

All these efforts to reduce overtreatment remind us that health-care costs are not on the rise because physicians are going around doing unnecessary heart transplants. Rather, it is the routine use of banal—and generally useless—tests and treatments that is costing us all a bundle. The researchers found, for example, that blood, urine and electrocardiogram tests are routinely ordered for patients with no related symptoms or risk factors. These are too often done merely to give a patient the sense that the doctor is "doing something."

Among the most frequently inappropriate practices Choosing Wisely identified were those that involved children with minor ailments: writing antibiotics prescriptions for children with sore throats who didn't have strep infection; recommending unnecessary cough syrup for children with upper respiratory infections; and ordering imaging tests such as computerized tomography (CT) scans for kids with minor head injuries (those that did not involve dizziness or loss of consciousness). Again, there are real, negative consequences to this kind of overtreatment, including fuelling antibiotic resistance and exposing people to potentially harmful radiation.

In Canada, we like to pretend overtreatment is a problem unique to the profit-driven US system, but we have many of the same problems. They are driven by bad habits more than by greed. North York General, a mid-sized hospital that has embraced Choosing Wisely, started by examining the wisdom of its everyday practices. It has about 100,000 emergency-room visits a year, and 42 percent of patients were getting at least one test (and often a battery of tests). After a review, that number dropped to 31 percent, and the top ten tests performed all dropped significantly in numbers. The result: shorter ER wait times for patients and savings of more than $150,000 for North York General. These initiatives initially focused on the blatantly wasteful, but now the hospital is beginning to tackle more controversial issues such as prostate-specific antigen (PSA) testing for prostate cancer and mass screening of young women for breast cancer. In those cases, the admonition is not for doctors to do nothing, but rather to be more targeted in their interventions. For some young women—those with several risk factors—early screening is appropriate. And for some men, the PSA test can be useful, as can surgery and/or radiation.

But watchful waiting also has its place. While that terminology has just recently come into vogue, there is an older term, *clinical inertia*, though it seems to have more negative connotations. For example, clinical inertia means having a patient with mildly elevated blood pressure or high cholesterol and deciding to not prescribe a drug. Instead, the doctor might encourage him to take a brisk walk each day or lose a few pounds, approaches that would be as effective as drugs and have no negative side effects. There was a time, not so long ago, when health professionals used this approach much more commonly, rather than immediately reaching for the prescription pad or the diagnostic test. Yet over time, physicians have been trained increasingly to become technicians and overly dependent on technology. Medicine is a science, but it is also an art. At its heart should be the art of listening, and the recognition that not acting is often as important as acting.

In the seminal work of satire *The House of God*, author Samuel Shem provided a list of commandments for good medical care. The infamous 13th Law of the House of God was, "The delivery of good medical care is to do as much nothing as possible." Yet, since the book's publication in 1978, overtreatment has reached such tragicomic proportions that the satire has melted away, leaving only age-old wisdom. It's as if we have come full circle back to Hippocrates, who said, "To do nothing is sometimes a good remedy."

If pot is medicine, treat it that way

It is estimated that there are now more than two hundred marijuana dispensaries across Canada—but that's just an educated guess because nobody's really counting. At first, they were most visible in

Vancouver, Victoria and Toronto, but now they are springing up just about everywhere. These dispensaries—which are illegal—are strange beasts: to purchase the products—dried, oil or edibles—you need a prescription for "medical" marijuana. Most dispensaries will refer you to a doctor who is happy to write a script for what ails you, such as pain (real or imagined). In Canada, if you have a prescription, you can also purchase medical marijuana directly from state-sanctioned suppliers and they will courier it to your home.

But now some dispensaries are not even bothering with the nudge-nudge, wink-wink of a prescription, selling pot to anyone who will sign a waiver saying they need it for medical reasons. These businesses are proliferating because of a grey zone created by the Liberal government's promise to legalize marijuana possession and its failure to provide concrete details on how it intends to do so.

The availability of drugs such as marijuana can be controlled in two basic ways: criminal prohibition and administrative regulation. Criminal prohibition has not worked—it has proven costly and ineffective. Pot is less harmful than tobacco or alcohol, but it is not benign. The best approach to reducing harm is to replace criminalization with health-focused regulation. This point was made eloquently by the Centre for Addiction and Mental Health in an October 2014 document titled *Cannabis Policy Framework*. The report makes a number of sound recommendations, including:

- setting a minimum age for cannabis purchase and consumption;
- limiting availability;
- curbing demand through pricing and taxation;
- curtailing higher-risk products and formulations;
- prohibiting marketing, advertising and sponsorship;
- clearly displaying product information, including labelling THC (tetrahydrocannabinol) and CBD (cannabidiol) content;
- addressing the risk of cannabis and impaired driving;
- enhancing access to treatment; and
- investing in education and prevention.

CAMH researchers also recommend, first and foremost, a government monopoly on sales of cannabis products.

But before blithely accepting dispensaries as a normal part of the urban landscape, we need to ask ourselves 1) whether marijuana is a legitimate prescription drug, and 2) whether stand-alone private businesses are the appropriate method for distribution of marijuana, "medical" or otherwise. A little bit of evidence (and, yes, plenty of anecdote) exists that marijuana is useful for treatment of some conditions, such as nausea and pain. But if cannabis is a legitimate prescription medicine, shouldn't it be subject to the same rules as other drugs, including being tested in clinical trials, packaged in measurable doses and sold in pharmacies? And why should we put conscientious physicians in the uncomfortable position of having to prescribe a sort-of-prescription drug that they know, in many cases, will actually be used for recreational purposes?

Canada has an estimated half a million users of "medical" marijuana over the age of twenty-five: 24,000 of them purchase the drug from state-approved suppliers, roughly 200,000 buy from grey-market dispensaries and almost 300,000 on the black market. Those numbers don't even include "recreational" users. Obviously, the time has come to fundamentally revamp our approach to pot. But public policy should be implemented deliberately and thoughtfully, not by pretending current regulations don't exist and allowing dubious approaches to fill the void. The move to legalization should be guided by public-health officials, not potpreneurs.

One of the key questions that flows from a promise of legalization is, where will marijuana be sold? Possible options are:

· in state-controlled outlets, the way beer and liquor is sold in many provinces;
· in corner stores, in the same way as cigarettes;
· in so-called coffee shops, as is done in the Netherlands; and
· in stand-alone dispensaries—with or without prescription.

What we have now is none of the above, with marijuana sold in unregulated, glorified head shops or by mail order. These approaches are, medically and legally, as preposterous as they are ridiculous.

The sale of marijuana is going to be legalized in Canada. The priority should be reducing harm, and the best way of doing so is with a state-controlled monopoly or, at the very least, firm regulation of private sales. We need to dispense with the Wild West of unregulated pot dispensaries. Canada needs to revamp its approach to pot, but public policy should be implemented deliberately and thoughtfully.

———⎍———

It's time to question the new cholesterol drug guidelines

According to 2013 guidelines published by the American Heart Association and the American College of Cardiology, every Caucasian male over the age of sixty-two, every African-American man over sixty-five, every white female over seventy, and every black female over sixty-nine should be taking statin medications, along with a whole bunch of younger people. In fact, the cardiology group believes one in every three adults needs these drugs to control their cholesterol levels. That beggars belief, considering there is little evidence statins prevent heart attacks and strokes in most people. It's no wonder these recommendations triggered a backlash and led to questions about whether cardiologists have put prescribing drugs ahead of preventing heart disease.

Most people of a certain age will know that it is fairly routine to have tests done to measure blood cholesterol levels. There is LDL, commonly referred to as bad cholesterol, and HDL, or good cholesterol. Ideally, you want to keep your LDL between 2.6 and 3.3 millimoles per litre, and HDL above 1.6 mml/L. (In the United States levels are measured in milligrams per decilitre—so you can multiply the Canadian numbers by forty.) At least, that has been the approach since guidelines were published in 2001, based on the assumption that reducing LDL and raising HDL would lower the risk of heart attack and stroke.

That approach is now being rejected. There is no longer a need to routinely monitor blood cholesterol, according to the 2013 guidelines. Why? Because the arbitrary cholesterol targets are not supported by scientific evidence. About three-quarters of people have normal cholesterol levels when they have heart attacks. That hasn't changed during the great statins experiment of the past decade and a half. Logically, this means physicians should be prescribing fewer statins, not more. But the newer guidelines have been sold as a "leap of faith," a belief that statins can prevent heart attacks and strokes, despite the fact that controlling cholesterol in otherwise healthy people has no such effect.

In brief, the research shows that statins are moderately effective in preventing heart attacks in men with a history of heart disease (meaning they've had a previous heart attack). They are not effective in women. And they don't provide much benefit, if any, to healthy people without a history of heart disease—regardless of their cholesterol levels. In fact, research published in October 2013 in the *British Medical Journal* by a group of researchers, including Dr. James Wright of BC's Therapeutics Initiative, found that 140 people would have to take statins for five years to prevent one heart attack. Further, about 18 percent of those taking statins suffer significant side effects, including diabetes, cataracts, liver damage and sexual dysfunction. Not to mention that the treatment costs about $1 a day per person—for life. That's pretty sobering data, particularly when you consider that 38 million prescriptions were filled for statins last year in this country.

Canada has not adopted the United States' latest cholesterol guidelines. The Canadian Cardiovascular Society said that the AHA/ACC guidelines were "not a game changer" but were "aligned" with the Canadian approach. What that means, in brief, is that Canadian cardiologists are still big believers in statins for controlling LDL/HDL levels and they think routine monitoring should continue.

Despite the growing evidence that statins are overused, the CCS is sticking to its guns: "The introduction of statins has created a paradigm shift for cardiovascular risk reduction, but there remains misunderstanding and fear of their use," they argue in the latest guidelines. Meanwhile, the US guidelines would actually result in more than doubling the number of people taking statins—from about 15 percent of adults currently to about one-third. Why? Well, according to the AHA and the ACC, they want physicians to focus on four groups who can most benefit from lowering LDL, or bad cholesterol, with statins, including:

· patients who have already been diagnosed with cardiovascular disease;
· people with very high LDL levels of 190 mg/dL or higher (4.9 mml/L in Canada), especially those with a genetic condition called familial hypercholesterolemia;
· everyone diagnosed with diabetes between the ages of forty and seventy-five; and
· all people aged forty to seventy-five who have a ten-year risk of cardiovascular disease of 7.5 percent or higher, based on a risk calculator that considers factors like age, weight and race.

The latter group is the most controversial. In earlier guidelines, patients were deemed to need statins if their risk of having a heart attack or stroke in the next decade was 20 percent or more. A lot of controversy has also arisen over the risk calculator itself because it's said to greatly exaggerate the risks. According to a commentary in the medical journal *The Lancet*, the calculator overpredicts the risk of a heart-related event by 75 to 150 percent. This has resulted in recommendations that virtually every senior citizen needs statins. That is clearly not the case.

Dr. John Abramson, a health policy lecturer at Harvard University, estimates that a person without existing cardiovascular disease can get as much benefit from a brisk daily ten-minute walk as from a daily statin pill—and without the potential side effects. Smoking cessation and weight loss would have even more dramatic effects.

Statins are not magical medications for prevention of heart disease. They give the illusion of protection. It is a costly illusion that needs to be shattered.

CHAPTER 4

War on Drugs

Hatred of supervised injection
sites is irrational

On September 21, 2003, Insite, Canada's only supervised injection
site, opened its doors. It began as a three-year research project
to determine if providing a safe place for intravenous drug users to
shoot up would help reduce the carnage on the streets of Vancouver's
Downtown Eastside. The idea was controversial then, and it's controversial now. In fact, if you look back at the clippings from 2003, you
quickly realize that the debate has not changed one iota in a generation,
at least at the emotional and political levels. Opponents say Insite
condones illicit drug use, encourages the congregation of unsavoury
characters and mollycoddles junkies instead of putting them in jail
where they belong. Proponents say that providing a place for addicts to
inject street drugs (heroin, cocaine, meth, opioids) with clean needles
is better than the alternative, having them share needles on the streets,
that it actually reduces criminal activity, and that mitigating the self-
harm of drug users is a better use of tax dollars than jailing them.

What has changed is the evidence, and the evidence shows that
Insite works. Overdose deaths from injectable drugs like heroin are
down, transmission of diseases like HIV-AIDS and hepatitis C among
users is down, drug-related crime in the area is down and use of addiction treatment services is up. While Insite is not solely responsible
for all these changes, it has played a role, particularly in the vulnerable
population of IV drug users.

Insite was never meant to be a panacea, a magic wand ending the scourge of drug addiction. A supervised injection facility is a harm-reduction measure and, bottom line, harm has been reduced. For that reason alone, public-health officials support supervised injection. Drug addicts are now shooting up in a facility dedicated to that purpose instead of doing so in back alleys, at the public library, in parks and in the washrooms at McDonald's. They are using clean needles instead of sharing. While getting their fix, addicts may get other medical care, reducing their need to go to the emergency room. Overdoses are now occurring where nurses are nearby to revive people (Insite has had nearly five thousand since it opened—roughly one a day among the eight hundred daily users—and not a single death) instead of those same overdoses happening on the streets and ambulance technicians rushing users to the ER, or the coroner having to come by and tag the body.

Should we be proud of the fact that there are thousands of addicts living on the streets of a wealthy Canadian city? Of course not. But we need to take measures that reduce the daily horrors of that reality. Public-health officials know that addiction is a sickness, not a crime. They are also a pragmatic lot; they take their victories, however small, wherever they can get them. And Insite's ongoing existence is, for the pragmatists, a big victory.

A comprehensive drug strategy needs four pillars: prevention, treatment, harm reduction and enforcement. For far too long, governments have put most of their eggs in the enforcement basket and neglected the others, and none more so than harm reduction. If harm reduction works—and it does—why don't we have supervised injection sites in Toronto and Montreal and Ottawa? And why don't we also invest in supervised inhalation sites, distribution of safe crack kits, and wet shelters? Why not find innovative ways to counter the scourge of methamphetamine and opioids addiction?

What we tend to get instead of practical, life-saving programs is a lot of moralistic lectures about the evils of addiction and the need to get "tough on crime." Government has a right to use the law to restrict the use of drugs, to declare them illicit and to impose sanctions on those who sell and use them. But government also has to recognize that you can't legislate away an illness like addiction, no matter how hard you try. Prevention and treatment (areas that are woefully neglected in our health-care budgets) and yes, even harm reduction, are all necessary components if we are going to have any hope of enforcement working.

The legal and political fights about Insite—and there have been many—should serve as a reminder that governments are supposed to be stewards, promoting the greater public good. They have a duty to act in ways that enhance the health of individuals and their communities, in a manner that is evidence informed, even when doing so is politically unpalatable and does not fit one's world view. The war-on-drugs mentality is not working. Isn't it time we used the insight gleaned from the Insite experience to create a smarter drug strategy?

Canada's pot policy needs to sober up

T he air is thick with pot talk in Canadian political circles these days, but the rhetoric is so extreme—ranging from "pot kills" to "pot cures cancer"—that it's sometimes hard to get a grip on what needs to be done. While the Liberal government has made it clear that smoking (or possessing) marijuana will no longer be a criminal offence, we do not yet know the precise details. Beyond decriminalization, there are also two distinct public-policy questions that need to be addressed:

· Is smoking marijuana safe and, if not, what should we do about it?
· Should marijuana be used as medicine?

Smoking is not healthy, regardless of what you smoke. But like other so-called recreational drugs, such as tobacco and alcohol, the risk is minimal with casual use. What matters is dose and frequency. A lot of Canadians smoke pot—about one in five currently and that would rise to one in three with decriminalization, polls show—but the vast majority do so in moderation. Marijuana is not addictive—in the common sense of the term, where stopping will cause withdrawal symptoms—though frequent users can become dependent, which is clearly not healthy. But our society has a lot more alcoholics than stoners.

Public-health authorities need to be pragmatic—to focus on harm reduction. That means warning people about the risks of marijuana smoking and especially about related activities, like the dangers of driving a motor vehicle or operating heavy machinery while stoned. And as with tobacco and alcohol, particular attention needs to be paid to young people and their developing brains. Excessive drug use, including marijuana, can affect learning and, in rare instances, be a trigger for more serious mental illness. What the public needs from health authorities is non-judgmental information, not *Reefer Madness* hysteria.

Without question, marijuana use has significant social and economic costs, most of it due to the criminalization of cannabis. Nearly eighty thousand Canadians a year are charged with marijuana-related offences, most of them for simple possession. It costs about $500 million a year to enforce our archaic marijuana laws, money that could obviously be spent better elsewhere. Having a criminal record is a lot worse for a person's health than smoking the occasional joint. Talking openly about marijuana use—and misuse—will certainly be easier when possession of small quantities of the drug is no longer a criminal offence. But there are still key details to be worked out, such as how much pot an individual can possess legally, how much it will be sold for (the retail price has to be lower than the street price) and where it will be sold. There will still be marijuana-related crimes, but they should not be an impediment to recreational users.

From a public-health perspective, a key question is whether decriminalization or legalization would incite more people to smoke marijuana. The polls suggest yes, but the experience from other jurisdictions shows the increase tends to be marginal. Examining the issue through a public-health lens, it is not logical to allow (and regulate and tax) the use of drugs like tobacco and alcohol and not do so with a drug that is no more harmful. The penalties for possession or use of marijuana are clearly out of whack with social norms.

The thorniest public-policy issue is so-called "medical" marijuana. About 24,000 Canadians now have a permit to purchase and use medical marijuana. Another 200,000 or so purchase "medicinal" pot from illegal but widely tolerated dispensaries. These "patients" smoke about four grams of pot a day, on average. There is a lot of anecdote and zeal about treating certain conditions—from cataracts to epilepsy—with marijuana. But the harsh fact is that not a lot of good scientific evidence exists that shows pot works systematically. The active ingredient in marijuana, THC, has potential. But no other drug is delivered by smoking. We don't have patients who need pain relief smoking opium, for example. We deliver opiates in controlled amounts with pills and injections. (Under previous rules, patients were allowed to grow their own pot, which was stranger still. Again, we don't have patients grow their own opium poppies.)

Of course, prescription drugs are not the be-all and end-all; they don't always work and they have side effects. A lot of Canadians also use so-called natural health products, and the evidence for their benefit is often scant. "Medical" marijuana's problem is that it is in a strange regulatory netherworld—it is neither a prescription drug nor a natural health product. Rather, we have a regulatory regime that requires physicians to approve access to marijuana (they don't actually prescribe) and the patient then orders it from a licensed supplier. The physician is a gatekeeper, with no intermediary like the pharmacist (or liquor store clerk) as there is with every other drug, prescription or otherwise. But physicians should not be policing marijuana use, no more than they police alcohol or tobacco use. To involve them gives marijuana a status it does not deserve.

Without the threat of legal action hanging over their heads, people could self-medicate with marijuana, just as they now do with Aspirin, St. John's wort and grandma's chicken soup. Prohibition doesn't work, especially for a drug that is widely used and has broad public tolerance. The marijuana policies we have in Canada are currently an asinine mishmash of repression and wishful thinking, and they need some serious revamping. Again, the obvious public-policy solution is decriminalization—but it has to be done right, with an eye to the implications for population health.

—⎯⌁⎯—

Sip on this: Like all drugs, alcohol isn't consequence free

Y ou can say this about Canadians: we like our beer. And wine, spirits and coolers. The average Canadian buys almost seventy-six litres of beer, sixteen litres of wine, five litres of spirits and four litres of other alcohol-based drinks annually. Alcohol is an accepted part of everyday life, a social lubricant at weddings, birthdays and parties, and a staple of sporting and cultural events, along with meals.

But there's a dark side to the $20.5 billion we spend annually on drink. Alcohol kills and maims in a perversely diverse number of ways, including liver disease, fetal alcohol spectrum disorder and impaired driving; it also fuels violence, sexual assault, suicide and traumatic injuries, and it hikes the risks of cancer and heart disease. All told, alcohol negatively affects more than two hundred health conditions. The impact of alcohol on health is one of the most neglected public-policy issues. That's why a 2015 report from Canada's chief public-health officer, Dr. Gregory Taylor, was a welcome, if long overdue, offering. The seventy-six-page report, titled *Alcohol Consumption in Canada*, presents some sobering statistics.

Alcohol is not a big killer, relatively speaking, accounting for about four thousand deaths a year in Canada, compared with thirty-seven thousand smoking-related deaths. (Marijuana activists will now chime in and remind us pot doesn't kill. Fair enough, though you can't entirely dismiss the harms of smoking pot.) In 2015, alcohol misuse cost the Canadian economy about $14.6 billion. About half that amount was lost productivity, with direct health-care costs estimated at $3.3 billion, and alcohol-related policing costs were not far behind at $3.1 billion. Motor vehicle crashes and fires related to alcohol cost another $1 billion a year. Meanwhile, alcohol sales and taxes bring in about $10.5 billion to state coffers.

A psychoactive substance, alcohol lowers inhibitions and impairs judgment. One of the most common and harmful side effects of overimbibing is violence—from bar fights to sexual assaults. More than one in three police calls are related to alcohol. Alcohol also has a direct impact on health. The ethanol in alcoholic drinks is particularly damaging to the liver, causing cirrhosis, but it is also carcinogenic, increasing the risk of everything from liver cancer to breast cancer. A depressant, alcohol can be particularly harmful to people with mental-health conditions such as depression. Almost one-third of people who die by suicide had been drinking excessively.

Still, alcohol is not all bad, nor should it be vilified. Most people drink responsibly, and moderate drinking—such as a glass of wine with dinner—can lower the risk of cardiovascular disease. In recent years, the number of abstainers has increased to about 20 percent of Canadians. (Worldwide, 60 percent of people do not drink, though it still kills about 3.1 million people a year; generally speaking, alcohol is consumed routinely in wealthy countries. Also, a number of religious prohibitions on alcohol exist.) But at the same time, the number of risky drinkers—defined at more than fifteen drinks weekly for a man or ten for a woman—and binge drinkers—those who drink to the point of blacking out or suffering alcohol poisoning—is on the rise, particularly among youth. Clearly, context matters a lot: how, where and when you drink has a significant influence on whether alcohol use is healthy or not.

One of the most troubling consequences of alcohol use and misuse is its impact on the fetus. In Canada, about three thousand babies a year are born with fetal alcohol spectrum disorder (FASD), and growing evidence suggests that even small quantities of alcohol can be damaging to the fetus. In February of 2016, the US Centers for Disease Control and Prevention found itself in hot water by recommending that women of childbearing age not drink unless they are using hormonal birth control because of the risk of FASD. While the message was well-intentioned—after all, half of pregnancies are not planned, and the damage done by alcohol is most pronounced in the first weeks when many women don't yet know they're pregnant—it was seen as condescending and paternalistic.

In short, as Taylor notes in his report, "the story of alcohol is complicated," and so is the necessary public-health response. History tells us that prohibition doesn't work. As with most public-health issues, the best tool is awareness—the recognition that, as with all drugs, recreational and medicinal, alcohol use and misuse is not consequence free.

---\|\---

The real opioid crisis is failed policy response

Opioid overuse is the worst man-made epidemic in modern medical history. We are creating a lost generation of people whose lives are being ruined by a rotating cast of opioid-based drugs: opium, cocaine, heroin, crack, OxyContin, fentanyl, carfentanil, W-18 and so on. The real crisis is not any particular drug, but our failed public-policy responses to drug use and abuse.

There always has been and always will be an appetite for the kind of escape and pain relief that drugs can provide, from alcohol through to W-18 and beyond. There has also long been a counter-vailing puritanical need to demonize pleasure and glorify suffering. Sure, drugs have the potential for harm, chief among them overdose and addiction. But most people who use drugs—even fentanyl—tend to do so responsibly, or at least how they're told to do so.

The worst consequences of drugs, those that are decried by political leaders and in newspaper headlines every day—like drug wars, criminality, violence, overdoses, the spread of infectious disease—are largely the result of criminalization (and to a lesser extent, misinformation), not drug use per se. They are self-inflicted wounds of prohibitionist policies. Cracking down on supply has never worked. We've known that at least since the Opium Wars in the nineteenth century. Yet we continue, futilely, to attempt to control supply, even as it gets ever easier to distribute drugs. You don't need a ship to move drug shipments anymore. Fentanyl doses are measured in micrograms; with one gram of base product, you can produce one thousand tablets. No border is tight enough to control the movement of drugs in the modern world, and no amount of policing will prevent people who want to use drugs from using them. So our aim should be responsible use.

Most users of opioids—up to and including fentanyl—are getting the drugs legally; they are being prescribed medication for the treatment of pain. The problem is that these drugs are overprescribed, particularly to those with chronic pain. A whopping 19.1 million opioid prescriptions were filled in 2015, making Canadians the world's biggest users per capita of narcotic painkillers. The number of people living with chronic pain is staggering—about one in five in the general population, and as many as three in five seniors. Yet the wait to be seen at a pain clinic can stretch for years, and the investment in physiotherapy and rehabilitation—alternatives to drugs—is paltry. So we drug people to a disturbing degree with often grim results: some get hooked and some overdose. The tragedy is that, while opioids are effective for cancer pain and in palliative care, they don't work for long-term chronic pain.

The issue of so-called recreational users of drugs is different. Many people from all walks of life (we're not sure how many because tracking illicit drug use is difficult) take opioids like OxyContin, heroin and fentanyl because it gives them a good buzz. They are occasional users. Then there is a small minority of opioid addicts, people we see living on the streets of our cities, big and small, and those who populate jails because of their drug crimes.

Addiction has many technical definitions, but a primary characteristic is persistence of use despite negative consequences. Locking up addicts isn't going to "fix" them. Criminalizing drug use, for addicts and occasional users alike, merely increases the risks. Users buy drugs of unknown quality and, when purchasing them illegally, put themselves at risk of physical and financial harm. The main reason people die from opioid overdoses is that the dose they took was greater than they believed, the drug was cut with harmful by-products and they were unable to get help.

There are an estimated two thousand opioid deaths a year in Canada (and another fourteen thousand in the United States). Most of the people dying are not street users but people introduced to the drugs medically, and legally. The single most effective way to reduce harm is to ensure these drugs are prescribed appropriately. We also need better education, for patients and medical practitioners alike, about the real benefits and risks of drugs like painkillers, investment in non-pharmaceutical pain-control methods, better access to addiction treatment, and harm-reduction measures.

In addition, we have to treat the most frightening symptoms of opioid use: overdoses. Naloxone (also known as Narcan) is a drug that has been used for decades in emergency rooms to reverse opioid overdoses. It blocks opiate receptors and essentially reverses the effects of drugs such as heroin. Naloxone should be as widely available as possible—carried by paramedics, police and firefighters and sold over the counter in pharmacies. The war-on-drugs folk think harm-reduction measures like naloxone aid and abet drug use. But we know that pragmatic harm-reduction measures are more effective than prohibition.

"Insanity," Albert Einstein is credited with saying, "is doing the same thing over and over again and expecting different results." For more than 150 years, we've been treating drug use, up to and including addiction, as a criminal matter rather than a public-health issue. It's well past time to concede that prosecution and persecution are poor substitutes for appropriate health and social services. We cannot arrest our way out of the opioids crisis.

CHAPTER 5

Aging

Stop blaming seniors for soaring health-care spending

I t is stated repeatedly—to the point that it has been accepted as fact—that the aging population is driving health-care costs through the roof. Aging baby boomers, we are told grimly, will bankrupt medicare. Bollocks.

What is true is that the number of seniors is rising—from 3.9 million in 2001 to an estimated 6.7 million in 2021, and 9.2 million in 2041. Put another way, the proportion of Canadians sixty-five and over will rise from 16 percent today to 25 percent as baby boomers age. It is also true that per-capita health spending—about $6,100 overall—increases markedly once people hit their so-called golden years: $6,298 for those aged sixty-five to sixty-nine, $8,384 for those seventy to seventy-four, $11,557 for those seventy-five to seventy-nine, and $20,917 for those eighty and older. Looking at those numbers, we assume, intuitively, that we are doomed. But let's not forget that seniors have been paying taxes their whole lives and the whole point of pooling money in a large public insurance plan is so the money is there when we need it, later in life.

The reality is that, whether you're four or forty or ninety, the majority of your lifetime health costs occur in the last year of life. But our health system has all kinds of cost drivers, and an aging population is only one of them. This point was made eloquently in a 2009 report from the Urban Futures Institute titled *Sustainable: British Columbia's*

Health Care System and Our Aging Population. While the report focuses on British Columbia, the messages are universal.

From 1979 to 2009, public spending on health care rose to $118.6 billion from $13.6 billion across Canada. In that same period, public spending in British Columbia jumped to $15.6 billion from $1.6 billion. (It has since risen to $160 billion nationally, and $18.5 billion in BC.) Four factors accounted for those increases:

- population growth—7 percent;
- aging of the population—14 percent;
- inflation—19 percent; and
- increased utilization—60 percent.

The Urban Futures analysis stated that the aging population is having an impact but, by far, what is driving health spending is utilization. We have new drugs, new technologies, new hospitals, more doctors and nurses (with higher incomes), new administrative structures and so on. Governments have been willing—save for a brief period in the early nineties—to increase health spending well above the rate of inflation with nary a concern.

During the thirty-year study period, health spending increased at an average rate of 8 percent a year. That is a much faster growth rate than inflation (3.4 percent), the over-sixty-five population (2.9 percent) and the general population (1.7 percent). Health spending has also, for three decades, grown faster than overall government spending (5.2 percent) and gross domestic product (5.3 percent). Still, some readers will say, "Sure, we've increased demand and costs, but seniors are the big users of care so it's their fault."

The Canadian Health Services Research Foundation, in its popular *Mythbusters* series, tackled the issue of aging seniors. It noted that over a generation, seniors have doubled their use of hospital and physician services, and their drug use has skyrocketed. The increases are much higher than in younger age groups. Why? Is the older-equals-sicker equation correct? Are twenty-first-century seniors really that much sicker than twentieth-century seniors? Or are we medicalizing aging to a perverse degree?

According to a fascinating article in the *Canadian Journal on Aging*, the cost of treating the sickest seniors—those in hospital—has remained relatively stable over a long period. On the other hand, the use of health services by healthy seniors (those who live independently in the community) has ballooned. Maybe all this extra spending is preventive and keeping people out of more expensive hospital care, though there is little concrete evidence of that. But there is a good deal of evidence that those with chronic illnesses—by far the biggest users of health services—are not being managed effectively or cost-efficiently.

Back to the Urban Futures report. It looked not only at trends thirty years back but offered projections thirty years forward. The authors estimate that, over the next three decades, as the influx of sixty-five-plus baby boomers comes and goes, state health spending will increase 84 percent—including 48 percent because of population growth and 36 percent because of the age composition of the population. In that same period, 2009 to 2039, GDP will grow an estimated 87 percent, meaning that, economically, we can easily handle the increased expense in health spending attributable to demographics. However, if utilization trends continue, health spending will increase an additional 191 percent and sustainability will be more precarious. To state it another way: for every $1 we spent in 2009, we will need $1.84 in 2039 to cover population growth and aging. But we will need $3.75 to keep pace if we continue with profligate shovelling of ever more tax dollars into sickness care well above the rate of inflation.

Canada's medicare system is not threatened by a silver tsunami of aging baby boomers. It is threatened by a tsunami of "more, more, more." It is threatened by an unwillingness to ask if more intense, more expensive care is appropriate or necessary, and a reluctance to reallocate dollars to strategies that work and to cut (or off-load) those that do not. Aging is inevitable, but thoughtless health inflation is not. So we should lay off the granny bashing and start making some tough choices.

We need a dementia strategy, not grandpa prisons

Like many who care for loved ones with Alzheimer's disease, Rose McLeod used visual clues to trigger memories. On the morning of September 2, 2010, she took out a wedding photo and marriage certificate to remind her husband of forty-eight years that they were indeed married. Joe McLeod responded angrily to the woman before him, convinced she was a stranger who had come into his home to do harm. Confused, he pushed her away brusquely. Rose fell to the ground; the framed wedding photo shattered and the glass cut her badly.

To this point, it is an all-too-common story, one that illustrates the challenges of caring for someone with dementia. A wedding photo, bloodied and in tatters, is poignantly symbolic. It is painful enough when someone you have loved for half a century no longer recognizes you. The paranoia and anger that are common in sufferers of Alzheimer's and some other forms of dementia make the pain more acute.

But Rose also suffered physical injury that day. She needed eight stitches to close the wound from the fall. In the emergency room, Rose recounted her ordeal with a mixture of sadness and exasperation. Police were called. Rose didn't want to press charges. Told it was the only way her husband could get help, she agreed, reluctantly. Joe McLeod, Alzheimer's patient, suddenly became Joe McLeod, wife beater. And this was where the story truly turned Kafkaesque.

Joe didn't get help. He spent more than a month in jail (the medical unit of the Winnipeg Remand Centre, to be more precise). He suffered a lot, scared and confused. That was because his wife, the person who cared for him around the clock, was forbidden from seeing him because she was considered a victim of domestic violence. On October 9, Joe was granted bail, and a bed was finally found for him in a long-term care facility. He would have spent even longer in the remand centre had his case not become a media *cause célèbre*. He still had to return to court to face a charge of assault causing bodily harm, but mercifully, charges were stayed. Later, Joe was moved to a care home, where he pushed a resident who died from his injuries. Joe was charged with manslaughter but found unfit to stand trial because of his dementia. He passed away in April of 2015.

Joe's story is not only a tragedy, it is a travesty of justice. It is also a graphic illustration of how the health system—and society more generally—is pathetically unprepared for the challenges posed by dementia, and psychiatric illnesses more generally. If the story of Joe McLeod sounds eerily familiar, it's because we have heard it so many times before. The loved ones of patients with psychiatric illnesses such as schizophrenia and bipolar disorder have lived these horrors—and these lies—for many years.

When a sick person urinates in public, shoplifts, trashes the family home or hits someone during a psychotic outburst, the police always say the same thing: press charges and they will get help. But the help too rarely comes. That's why our prisons are full of people with mental illness. (One in eight federal prisoners has a diagnosable mental illness, and the rate is significantly higher in provincial jails.) All we need now is to start dispatching elderly Alzheimer's patients to jail for their transgressions.

Let's state it plainly so that politicians, judges, physicians and others in positions of responsibility understand: it is unacceptable to jail someone with Alzheimer's. Psychosis is a common symptom of Alzheimer's and other forms of dementia. It needs to be treated, not punished. Jail is not—and will never be—a substitute for care, and care should never be dependent on criminal charges. Our health system and our justice system need to be more humane and rational than that. We don't need grandpa prisons. We need a dementia strategy.

Health authorities' lack of planning and failure to take this issue seriously were the real reasons Rose ended up in the emergency room with serious injuries. She had been caring for her husband for more than two years as his mental and physical condition deteriorated steadily. (Joe also had serious heart disease.) Before the incident occurred, he'd begun to wander and required around-the-clock care. Rose didn't receive the training and education that would have helped her prepare for the predictable outbursts of violence. Her attempts to find a long-term care home for her husband were unsuccessful. She didn't get home care to help her cope with escalating demands. No one was there to help the family navigate the complex health, legal and social welfare systems. The painful shove from her husband was the least of the assaults Rose had to endure. That the same system that failed to help her was all too willing to incarcerate a sick man for being sick added insult to injury.

According to Alzheimer's Society Canada, in 2016 an estimated 564,000 Canadians were living with dementia, with about 25,000 new cases diagnosed every year. By 2031, that number is expected to rise to 937,000, an increase of 66 percent. There are about 3.8 million informal caregivers in Canada—people caring for their loved ones with dementia and other debilitating illnesses. It is in the interests of these patients, and of society more generally, that they live at home as long as possible. For this to happen, caregivers need help—from home-care workers, system navigators and public-policy changes. They also need the assurance that, when the time is right, a bed will be available in a long-term care facility.

Joe was asked by Judge Sandra Chapman if he would comply with his bail conditions. "I will do my best," he said. If only the legal and health systems would vow to do the same for the over half-million other Canadians who suffer from dementia.

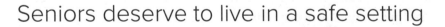

Seniors deserve to live in a safe setting

Just after midnight on January 23, 2014, a blaze broke out in the kitchen of the Résidence du Havre nursing home in L'Isle Verte, Quebec. Thanks to the inept response that followed, thirty-two seniors—who had moved to an institutional setting in order to be safe and cared for—died horrific deaths. The orgy of inaction and excuse-making that followed suggests we have learned nothing from this preventable tragedy.

An extensive police investigation was held, but no criminal charges were laid. These deadly fires happen all too often, but no one ever seems to be responsible. Yet in his report, coroner Cyrille Delâge was scathing in pointing out that there was plenty of blame to go around. Initially, fingers were pointed at ninety-six-year-old Paul-Étienne Michaud, an occasional smoker. But crime scene investigators found that the fire started in the kitchen just below Michaud's room and he was, in fact, the first victim.

Just a single worker was responsible for the overnight care of the fifty-two residents of the nursing home, even though most were over eighty-five and suffering from mobility and cognitive challenges. The actions of that employee, Bruno Bélanger, on the fateful night were head-scratchingly bizarre. After the fire started, he ran past the rooms of at least a dozen residents without notifying them, saying he was in a rush to get to the room of his employer/girlfriend at the opposite end of the complex, because that was "protocol." Bélanger had never participated in a single fire drill and said he didn't even know how to operate a fire extinguisher, even though he had been a fire-extinguisher salesman for fifteen years—a palpable irony.

The front door of the nursing home was locked and could not be opened from the inside. Several bodies were found there; most others were found on balconies, where residents prayed and screamed for help that did not come fast enough. The bodies were so badly burned that they had to be identified by the serial numbers on their artificial hips and false teeth. It took eighteen minutes for volunteer firefighters to arrive on the scene, and the fire chief did not call in reinforcements until nineteen minutes after he arrived on site; the closest professional firefighting crew, in Rivière-du-Loup, was never called. Once again, the excuse was "protocol." It turned out that most of the firefighters didn't have proper training either; the municipality said it didn't want to impose on volunteers.

The most disturbing contributing factor to the tragedy, however, was that no sprinkler system was installed in the part of the building where everyone died, something that provincial regulators tried to defend with Byzantine and bureaucratic explanations that made Delâge explode with anger. "The law should be simple and straightforward: every institutional facility like a nursing home should have an automatic sprinkler system. Period." Delâge first made that recommendation in 1969, when he conducted an inquest into the Repos du Vieillard nursing home fire in Notre-Dame-du-Lac that killed thirty-eight seniors.

Since then, too many similar tragedies with mass casualties have occurred, including the Chafe's Nursing Home fire in Petty Harbour, Newfoundland, on Boxing Day 1976 that left twenty-one people dead, and the 1980 fire at the Extendicare home in Mississauga that claimed the lives of twenty-five seniors. And that is without mentioning the incidents that occur all too often that claim "only" a couple of lives.

How much more carnage do we need before taking decisive action? Canada has more than 400,000 Canadian seniors living in institutional settings, and they deserve to be safe. We have a national fire code—it says sprinklers should be mandatory in every institutional residence—but most provinces have not made that recommendation law. And even the jurisdictions that have mandated the installation of sprinklers have grandfather clauses (a particularly egregious expression in this instance) for existing facilities and lag times of up to a decade for retrofitting. In Quebec, for example, fewer than half of the nursing homes have sprinkler systems. It is cold comfort to know that granny's old-age home will finally be fitted with twentieth-century safety equipment some time before 2025.

As Coroner Delâge is fond of saying, "The best way to fight fires is with prevention." But there have been far too many inquiries, and far too little action has been taken on their recommendations. The words *patchwork* and *bureaucracy* are being used a lot to describe the regulatory environment that is supposed to keep our elders safe. *Contemptuous* would be more precise.

Our elderly are adrift in a sea of drugs

In 2004, the quirky, popular syndicated column "The Straight Dope" examined the legend that the "Eskimos" put their old people on ice floes and set them adrift. The writer suggested that senilicide (the killing of old people) did occur during severe famines, but the last recorded case was in 1939, and even before that it was a rarity. "The common perception of taking granny out to the nearest ice floe and setting her adrift is wrong."

But the common belief that granny is a lot better off today than in the mythically cruel Arctic of old may be equally wrong. In fact, there is ample evidence that senilicide is more common in our wealthy, modern Canadian society than it ever was in Inuit society. We don't set our elders adrift on ice floes, but we do the modern equivalent: we drug them into icy oblivion.

Seniors take a mind-boggling number and variety of drugs. According to the Canadian Institute for Health Information, two-thirds of Canadians over sixty-five have five or more different prescriptions, and one-quarter take ten or more prescription drugs. The older you get, the more drugs you take. More than 40 percent of advanced seniors (eighty-five and older) take ten or more drugs. In institutionalized care, nursing homes or long-term-care facilities, the numbers are even higher. It is not unusual for patients to have twenty to twenty-five prescriptions, their lives a non-stop ritual of pill-popping and trying to manage the side effects.

The sheer quantity of drugs prescribed is alarming, but the way some drugs are used is even more disturbing. Almost half of seniors in long-term care are prescribed antipsychotics, and 20 percent take them chronically. For the most part, these drugs are prescribed "off-label," not because people are psychotic but to calm them or help them sleep. Dementia patients in hospitals and nursing homes are routinely chemically restrained—sedated, if you prefer—to protect them from harming themselves and others. This practice is fuelled by the myth that people with dementia are violent; in fact, many are agitated and lash out because they are confused and frightened. Understaffing and our disdain for aging and the elderly lead us to opt for drugging over other, more hands-on approaches to care.

In 2014, John Wright, then-president and CEO of the Canadian Institute for Health Information, told the Senate Committee on Social Affairs, Science and Technology that Canadian data show that at least one in ten seniors is taking a prescription drug that is "potentially dangerous." While drugs have benefits, they also have side effects, particularly when they interact, when they are taken in the wrong doses or when the wrong drug is prescribed. About 10 percent of all admissions to hospital among seniors are due to reactions to drugs. In fact, seniors are five times more likely to be hospitalized for adverse drug reactions than non-seniors. To compound the problem, misuse of drugs also occurs frequently in hospitals. A landmark 2004 report on "adverse events" (also known as medical errors) found that between 9,250 and 23,750 Canadians die annually because of these avoidable errors in hospitals. Most of the deaths were among seniors—the principal clientele of hospitals—and almost half were drug-related. Of course, all this prescribing is well-intentioned—but so was setting people on an ice floe. It does not excuse the dreadful outcomes.

Aside from the obvious waste of money in a cash-strapped system—money that could be better spent providing seniors with services they desperately need, such as home care—there is very little tracking of the appropriateness or inappropriateness of prescription drugs.

Thankfully, the tide is beginning to turn. There is a growing recognition that the number of drugs we pump into seniors is madness. The Canadian Deprescribing Network has set the lofty goal of reducing unnecessary and inappropriate medication use in seniors by 50 percent by 2020. The initiative is part of a growing and welcome trend to question the "more is better" approach to medicine. To begin with, it is focusing on classes of medication that are the most overused, misused and potentially harmful, such as benzodiazepines (sedatives to help people sleep) and proton pump inhibitors (used to treat heartburn, but which raise the risk of fractures and infections).

Hopefully, they will also move quickly to promote deprescription of opioid-based painkillers; while overdose-related deaths have generated a lot of media interest in recent years, it is often forgotten that most of these deaths are due to prescribed medications, not street drugs, and the most common victims are seniors. And of course, ensuring that prescriptions for antipsychotics are appropriate should be a priority.

As the Senate committee noted in its 2014 report, virtually no cost-benefit analyses are done on prescribing practices, and very little follow-up is done on how individuals—and seniors in particular—fare. Without this information, without these checks and balances, our elders are being cast adrift, not on an ice floe, but in a pharmacological haze.

CHAPTER 6

End of Life

Whose life is it anyway?

" **I** f I cannot give consent to my own death, whose body is this? Who owns my life?" Sue Rodriguez famously asked. In 1993, the Supreme Court of Canada rejected her bid to strike down the Criminal Code provisions making assisted suicide a crime, in large part because the prohibition was deemed to be consistent with Canadian values. Eventually, Rodriguez got her assisted death—albeit not legally. And over the next two decades, her whispered question rumbled just below the surface. As baby boomers aged, values changed. So did expectations. But Canada's laws, and its lawmakers, did not keep pace.

But in 2014, death came out of the closet. The end-of-life conversation, which for so long was conducted in apprehensive, hushed tones, grew boisterous, and the "death with dignity" debate took centre stage in the mainstream media, various legislatures and even the Supreme Court of Canada. One of the most poignant contributions to the debate came from Gillian Bennett, an eighty-three-year-old woman in the early stages of dementia who posted a farewell letter on her blog, Dead at Noon, before lying down on the beach near her home on Bowen Island, BC, and taking a fatal dose of barbiturates.

Kim Teske, suffering from the degenerative Huntington's disease, chose a different tack, starving herself to death to protest the absurdity of Canadian laws that don't allow for assisted death. Margot Bentley, a former nurse with dementia, thought she had done everything right by stating in her will that she wanted to refuse all treatment, but she ended up being force-fed because the courts ruled that is not a medical intervention. Hamilton journalist Eric McGuinness, an outspoken right-to-die activist who suffered from terminal cancer, travelled to Zurich to end his life legally there. In an earlier essay, McGuinness said, "I want to die as easily and humanely as a loved family pet."

What all those *cris de coeur* had in common was a demand by dying people to have their end-of-life wishes respected. They also added human faces and a sense of urgency to a case that had taken many years to work its way to the Supreme Court. Others included Gloria Taylor, who suffered from ALS (also known as Lou Gehrig's disease) and wanted an assisted death but was denied one, and Kay Carter, who suffered from spinal stenosis and also opted for assisted death in Switzerland. They became the central figures in the drama even though both had died by the time the legal battle reached the top court.

On February 6, 2015, the Supreme Court struck down two sections of the Criminal Code: Section 14 stated that "no person is entitled to consent to have death inflicted upon them," and Section 241(b) stated that anyone who "aids or abets a person to commit suicide" commits a crime. The court further stated that patients who are "grievously and irremediably" ill have the constitutional right to choose hastened death. It was a watershed moment. But the court also gave the federal government a year to fashion new legislation. The government of Stephen Harper, in power at the time, was firmly opposed to assisted death, so it chose to do nothing other than to appoint a panel to study the issue—the External Panel on Options for a Legislative Response to Carter v. Canada. The provinces appointed their own study group, the Provincial-Territorial Advisory Group on Physician-Assisted Dying.

Creating a law that pleased everyone was impossible. Staunch objections came from religious groups, some disability activists and palliative-care providers. Civil libertarians demanded that government get out of the way, that legislation was not even necessary. (Canada's abortion law was declared unconstitutional by the Supreme Court in 1988; legislators were never able to agree on a new law, so provision of the service was guided by ethical rules of health professionals rather than statute, an approach that worked out fine.) Meanwhile, regulatory bodies for health-care workers like physicians, nurses and pharmacists had to create constitutionally valid, medically responsible guidelines, and along with hospitals and nursing homes, had to prepare for the practicalities of providing consent forms, formulations for lethal cocktails, and billing codes.

In the end, Bill C-14, Medical Assistance in Dying, was adopted on June 17, 2016. It is a disappointing law because it establishes rules for assisted death that are far more restrictive than those set out by the Supreme Court. The most controversial aspect of the federal law is the criterion that a person's death must be "reasonably foreseeable" for them to be eligible for assisted death. That term, which is not defined, has no legal or medical meaning. The legislation also makes it nearly impossible for patients with dementia or those suffering from mental illness to be granted assisted death because it does not allow advance consent, and it limits requests to those over the age of eighteen, although mature minors can make decisions on all other medical treatments.

Bill C-14 may well be unconstitutional. At the very least, it will result in many more years of costly and unnecessary court challenges. The law is far from perfect. In a very short time, assisted death went from being a crime to being a right. Canadians—or at least many Canadians—can now choose how they die, and they can die with a little more dignity.

--\|--

Armed with the principles, on to the practicals

The Supreme Court of Canada, in lifting the legal impediments to physician-assisted death, expressed clearly what most Canadians believe: that denying a hastened death to those who are suffering "intolerably and permanently" is cruel. Denying them the choice is also unconstitutional. The learned justices acknowledged that if a person of sound mind and failing body chooses to die, she or he should be able to do so humanely, with the aid of a physician or nurse practitioner, and not have to leap from a balcony, poison themselves with pills or flee to a country such as Switzerland for a life-ending cocktail.

But since the day of that historic judgment, February 6, 2015, the challenge has been to give the ruling life. The decision may have been two decades in the making, but the debate has only just begun. Technically, the ruling, known as Carter v. Canada, struck down two sections of the Criminal Code that made assisting suicide, or asking someone to assist in your death, a crime. But in practice, it set off a cascade of legal requirements for the federal government, provincial and territorial governments, and regulatory bodies. It also gave both proponents and opponents of assisted death new ammunition and helped establish new battle lines.

First of all, the federal government had to pass legislation (or not) to replace the parts of the Criminal Code that were struck down. Assisting suicide remains a crime in Canada, but the new law provides an exemption for physicians and nurse practitioners if they respect a series of conditions. These include a provision that the death of the person making the request is "reasonably foreseeable"—meaning, presumably, that they don't have long to live but are suffering unduly. The law also requires that two physicians sign off on the request, and that a cooling-off period of ten days be respected to ensure the person is serious about the request (though the wait can be shortened in some circumstances).

However, a law has to be fleshed out with regulations, and their formulation is a tedious, technical process that can take up to two years. Legislators must, for example, set out the penalties for violating the law (a conviction of assisting suicide can result in a prison term of up to fourteen years). Ottawa also has an essential role in monitoring compliance with the law. But in the absence of regulations about what exactly physicians, hospitals and provinces/territories have to report, there is a lot of confusion and frustration in the field. Monitoring is crucial to understanding who is requesting assisted death, who is undergoing the procedure, and who is being refused. If you want to know whether the law is working—whether the court ruling is being respected—you have to study how it's being applied.

Under Canada's constitutional regime, provinces are responsible for the delivery of care and for other areas like insurance. So, for example, each province and territory needs to pass legislation stating specifically that people who opt for assisted death cannot be denied life insurance payouts (because many insurance contracts have a clause denying payment in the case of suicide). Provinces also have to decide if drugs used for assisted death—usually a cocktail of three drugs: a benzodiazepine, a calming sedative; then a barbiturate to induce a coma; and finally, a neuromuscular blocking agent that causes the heart and lungs to stop—are covered by provincial health plans. (Drugs usually are covered in hospital, but not outside.) They need to decide whether the lethal drug has to be administered by a physician or nurse, or whether it can be self-administered. They also have to create billing codes so health practitioners can be reimbursed for the medical act, and design formularies to track assisted deaths and those that are refused.

The Supreme Court ruled that physicians, nurses and other health workers cannot be compelled to participate in assisted death, that they have a right to conscientious objection. But provinces and territories have to decide if that opt-out can extend to institutions. Most faith-based institutions, both hospitals and nursing homes, have said they will not provide assisted death. Many palliative-care facilities—and even palliative-care units in public hospitals—have also taken a hard line. But right-to-die activists argue that any facility that receives public funding has an obligation to provide this medically necessary service and that transferring patients who are already suffering at the end of life to "non-objecting" facilities is unnecessarily cruel.

Federal legislation features an unusual requirement for a parliamentary review within five years. That's because legislators recognize there is a lot of unfinished business. The most contentious debate of all revolves around who is eligible—and ineligible—for assisted death. Allowing adults who are terminally ill and in their final days or weeks of life but still of sound mind to opt for assisted death is easy, relatively speaking. But what about children, people with dementia and those with severe mental illness? How do you judge if they're competent and able to make rational decisions? If you have more liberal rules, how do you prevent the vulnerable—the frail elderly, people with severe mental and physical disabilities, and those with dementia—from being pressured into hastening their deaths?

Those lines can be blurry. Those debates can be intense. Already, the constitutionality of the law is being challenged by those who want people in the early stages of dementia to be able to give prior consent to assisted death when their condition deteriorates. That won't be an easy decision to make for the courts or for legislators. But eventually, decisions will have to be made—tough decisions. Hopefully, they will be made promptly and thoughtfully.

It's not enough to have laws saying patients have a right to assisted death. Physicians, institutions and lawmakers must ensure that the right can be exercised in a timely, fair and ethical way.

—/\—

The language of life, the language of death

I n matters of life and death, words matter. As the public discussion about end-of-life issues has become more commonplace and more nuanced, the vocabulary has become more sophisticated.

In 2012, Gloria Taylor, who suffered from amyotrophic lateral sclerosis, won the right, in BC's Supreme Court, to end her life at the time of her choosing. She argued that, because of the physical limitations caused by ALS, she was unable to take her own life (which is legal) and therefore entitled to the assistance of a physician to help by administering a death-hastening drug. The landmark case—which eventually worked its way up to the Supreme Court and resulted in sections of the Criminal Code being struck down—landed the story on the front pages of newspapers and at the top of broadcasts.

But journalists had a dilemma: What do you call the right Taylor won? Physician-assisted suicide? Physician-enabled death? Physician-hastened death? Euthanasia? Voluntary euthanasia? Rational suicide? Suicide? Mercy killing? State-sanctioned murder? Death with dignity? And there are many more variations, each loaded with legal and moral baggage. The language we choose tends to reflect where we stand on the underlying question of whether grievously and irremediably ill people should have the right to choose to end their lives rather than let an illness take its course.

Ultimately, the fundamental legal issue is choice: Do individuals have control over their bodies in death as in life? Those who are pro-choice use neutral language like "medical aid in dying" or "medical assistance in dying" (the terminology eventually used in Quebec legislation and federal legislation, respectively) and describe their quest as ensuring death with dignity. Those who are anti-choice use more loaded terms like "assisted suicide" and "euthanasia."

But suicide is an act of self-harm that is often a by-product of mental illness like schizophrenia or severe depression. That is in no way comparable to hastening death via a methodical, sober process with a number of legal safeguards. Calling medically assisted dying suicide is a lot like calling surgery a knife attack. *Euthanasia* is similarly rife with negative implications. The word's origin is found in the Greek prefix *eu*, meaning "good," and *thanatos*, meaning "death," so it means a "quiet and easy death." But the term was forever perverted by the Nazis, who used *euthanasia* to describe some of their murderous atrocities.

This provides a good segue into discussing the greatest fear about legalizing (or more precisely, decriminalizing) medical assistance in dying—that it will throw open the door to abuse, to euthanasia of the frail, sick elderly and those with disabilities. We already have a word for the practice: murder. In contrast, physician-assisted death has to be consensual, and it is only appropriate in a limited number of cases—those of patients who are grievously and irremediably ill. (In everyday language we would say "terminally ill," but that term is imprecise. Unfortunately, the language that ended up in federal law, "reasonably foreseeable death" is equally imprecise.)

For a long time, it was difficult for those who choose to end their lives to do so in a dignified manner. The political and legal climate encouraged secrecy, isolation and underground practices, and many families and physicians harbour painful secrets because they fulfilled the final wish of a loved one. In reality, even before medical assistance in dying became legal in June 2016, there had been plenty of assisted deaths already. The subtle but important difference is that intervention was passive rather than active—and, in fact, the former continues to be much more common than the latter.

There is "withdrawing of potentially life-sustaining treatment"— also crudely called "unplugging a patient"—when patients with no hope of recovery are mercifully removed from respirators that are keeping them alive artificially. Another common practice is "palliative sedation," gradually jacking up the dose of pain medication to ease suffering, which usually leads to respiratory failure. Not to mention what health-care practitioners call VSED (voluntary stopping of eating and drinking), when terminally ill patients refuse food and drink (or their substitute decision-makers do so on their behalf), essentially starving themselves to death with the compassionate complicity of their care providers.

These practices are not wrong; quite the opposite. Optimal medical care, especially at the end of life, is about relieving pain and suffering, not keeping someone nominally alive at all costs. Caring physicians should not be reduced to doing so in a nudge-nudge, wink-wink fashion. Too often, we see death as a failure of medicine and inflict all manner of so-called heroic interventions on patients who really need palliative care and, in some instances, a helping hand in bringing an end to their suffering. Death is part of the cycle of life. We should not fear it, but plan for it. That includes making our personal wishes explicit, with living wills and in frank discussions with our loved ones, and we need to do so using words that are precise and meaningful, not euphemistic. We need to give life to the language of death.

CHAPTER 7

Children

Our schools shape kids' minds
but neglect their bodies

School is a place to learn, to play, to make friends, and for stolen first kisses. School is where children learn to become independent from their parents, where they shape their values and forge their links to the community, and where the seeds of their future careers are sown. School is a place where lifelong habits, good and bad, are formed. As such, we owe it to ourselves and to our children to make schools as safe and healthy as possible.

But schools are failing the health test. They don't pay adequate— or the right kind of—attention to the well-being of the country's 5.5 million primary and secondary students. School safety is all too often equated with keeping out maniacal gunmen and sexual predators. What should concern parents more than these extreme and rare threats are the mundane realities of everyday school life—the physical environment, the safety of transport, the food that is consumed, the activity that is (and is not) undertaken and the health lessons that are taught, both explicitly and implicitly.

The most hazardous part of a student's day, by far, is the trip to school. Children travel by bus, by car and occasionally by foot, braving encounters with the primary killer of kids, the motor vehicle. Those in buses have the added disadvantage of being transported in vehicles not equipped with seat belts.

Children spend at least six hours a day in school, and it's not unusual for the day to stretch to ten hours or more with before- and after-school care and activities. In fact, for ten months a year, during the most formative years of their lives, children and youth spend the bulk of their waking hours in educational institutions. Yet parents know remarkably little about the surroundings in which they learn and the curriculum they are taught. Every child receives a report card, yet schools themselves are not systematically graded. The evidence is anecdotal, but many schools are old and have poor air quality and mould. Many were built in an era when lead pipes and asbestos were staples of construction; too many fail to meet modern fire-safety norms. A lot of schools are overcrowded and poorly ventilated, making them hotbeds for disease transmission. Outbreaks of meningitis, whooping cough, chickenpox and influenza are still too common. Vaccination is not always mandatory and even when it is, the rules are rarely enforced. Significantly, classrooms themselves tend to be ergonomic wastelands. As if the packsacks they lug around are not damaging their backs enough, children often sit at desks and on chairs that are uncomfortable and backbreaking.

And sit they do. The vast majority of schools in Canada do not offer daily physical activity as part of the curriculum, and where they do it is often a tedious ritual of standing around. Gym class should be about planting a seed so that physical activity becomes part of their lifestyle as children grow up, yet there is, on average, only six minutes of actual movement in a typical gym class. Playgrounds, if they exist at all, tend to be rickety. And how many schools have anything but asphalt yards? After hours, school gyms are often locked up tight or charge exorbitant fees, making them inaccessible. Prisoners get more daily activity and often have better recreational equipment and freer access to facilities than children in public schools.

And what about the food? The staple of many school cafeterias remains hot dogs and fries. Vending machines loaded with sugary and salty snacks are ubiquitous. While that's changing, Canada remains the only G8 country that does not have extensive school-based feeding programs.

Children and teens should be getting the tools that allow them to build and maintain a healthy lifestyle. They need education about fitness, nutrition and sexual health to be integrated into every aspect of the curriculum, not tossed in as an afterthought as part of the dreaded lectures from the gym teacher about the birds and the bees. Children also need role models and inspiring surroundings. They need to see good health and fitness valued. Yet most schools do not even have a school nurse anymore, so health promotion has fallen by the wayside. We cannot expect to produce healthy adults if we lock them into unhealthy institutions for the thirteen years of their primary and secondary education.

Then there is homework—a largely counterproductive time suck. For more than seventy years, research has demonstrated that the more kids play, the better they learn. In fact, a landmark study conducted in 1951 in Vauves, France, found that the school day that maximizes learning consists of two-thirds classroom time, one-third physical education—and no homework so kids can play more (and not video games). That research has been replicated many times, with slight permutations but the same results. The obsession with test scores has not produced smarter children, but it has produced more unhealthy ones. We are wasting tremendous opportunities by focusing singularly on the three Rs and failing to educate our children properly about healthy living.

Healthy schools are not a luxury, they are a necessity. The learning environment we create is fundamental to our social and economic well-being, a key to future productivity and the sustainability of the health-care system. We cannot expect academic success and innovation in environments that are poisonous. We cannot afford to focus so exclusively on children's academic studies that their physical, mental and emotional health is laid to waste. We cannot produce healthy citizens if our schools and our approaches to learning are unhealthy.

Decades later, lead is still
stalking our kids

Getting the lead out of our environment has been one of the notable public-health success stories of the past generation. Thirty years ago, lead, a heavy metal that is toxic even at low levels—and especially to children—was ubiquitous. It was used as an additive in gasoline, as solder in canned goods, paints, water pipes, fishing lures and sinkers and even in pencils. Today, almost all those uses have been phased out. But the cover story in the April 2005 edition of *Nutrition Action Healthletter*, the consumer magazine published by the Center for Science in the Public Interest in the United States, serves as a reminder that lead, and its attendant health risks, is still with us in many ways. Over a decade later, the issues remain, and interest has been revived by the Flint, Michigan, water crisis, where cost-cutting measures resulted in residents being exposed to lead and other toxins in their drinking water.

In the United States, more than 500,000 children suffer from lead poisoning every year—most of them in low-income neighbourhoods in Rust Belt cities. A 2013 study showed that in Baltimore alone, 65,000 children had dangerously high lead levels in their blood. Research published over the past few decades has demonstrated that virtually everyone over the age of forty-five has significant quantities of lead accumulated in their bones. According to Health Canada, in 1979, 27 percent of Canadians had lead levels in their blood exceeding ten parts per million, or ten micrograms per decilitre; today about 1 percent of Canadians do. But that is still a significant number—360,000 people—especially when you consider that there is no safe level of lead exposure. (The us Centers for Disease Control and Prevention says levels of more than five parts per million pose a significant health risk, especially for children.) Unfortunately, very little investigation about who is at risk, and why, is being done in Canada.

Lead has a half-life of about twenty-five years in bones, meaning it takes that long for our bodies to purge just half the amount that has accumulated. As baby boomers age, this continued presence of lead—a neurotoxin that damages the brain—becomes an ever-growing risk because it seems to accelerate and worsen many of the health conditions associated with aging—namely, osteoporosis, hypertension, diabetes, Alzheimer's and other forms of dementia. Research published in the *Journal of the American Medical Association* showed that people with high lead levels in their bones scored consistently lower on tests of memory and mental agility. One study estimated that a high lead level translated to three to six years of aging of the brain. Research has also demonstrated that people with high lead levels are about three times more likely to develop cataracts, a serious eye disease linked to hypertension and calcium levels. The danger is particularly great to menopausal women. As bones thin and lose calcium and other minerals, lead is released into the bloodstream at a faster rate. The long-term Nurses Health Study showed that lead levels increased 25 to 30 percent after menopause, even though heavy exposure stopped decades earlier, and that high levels of lead in the blood may even trigger early menopause.

Research conducted on US veterans found that those with the highest level of lead in their bones were twice as likely to have high blood pressure as those with low levels. Researchers at the Harvard School of Public Health found that even modest amounts of lead in the body led to significant deterioration of kidney function, particularly in people with underlying renal problems. For example, the effect of lead on the kidneys was about fifteen times greater for patients with diabetes.

In addition to cataloguing the health risks from accumulated lead among people of a certain age, the article in *Nutrition Action Healthletter* also serves as a reminder that many consumers are still unwittingly being exposed to lead. Most homes built before 1950 have lead water pipes and/or lead service lines bringing in water from the street. Until two decades ago, lead was still used to solder brass and copper pipes. Many homes built before 1976 have lead-based paints, a health risk when they chip or peel. The advocacy group Environmental Defence Canada estimates that about 15 percent of Canadian homes still have worrisome lead levels, principally from drinking water. You can minimize your risk by running the water before drinking it, by using cold water for cooking (hot water leaches more lead) and by installing a filter. You can also test your drinking water for lead, cheaply and easily.

Baby boomers should be concerned with the impacts of lead on their own health, but they should not forget that their grandchildren are also at risk. Despite an over forty-year crackdown, lead is probably still the foremost environmental health risk to Canadian children. Lead poses a real danger to developing brains and nervous systems, and even non-toxic levels of exposure can take several points off a child's IQ. Yet lead is still used in the PVC blinds that are commonplace in Canadian homes, although Health Canada recommends they be removed from all homes with children under the age of six. Cheap, dollar-store jewellery has been found to contain high lead levels, and sometimes so have crayons. So does makeup. Continuing industrial emissions mean that most foods contain trace amounts of lead. Many children are also exposed to lead in soil when they play in the dirt, as well as to lead in paint and drinking water. By some estimates, as many as one in five children today has worrisome lead levels in his or her blood; this shows that lead remains quite pronounced in their environment.

So while superficially at least, measures to reduce lead in the environment—such as banning leaded gasoline and lead-based paints— have been successful from the public-health side, the ongoing story is a stark reminder that when we do tackle complex environmental and public-health challenges, the results are not always immediate and are rarely universal, and the fallout can be unpredictable. The need for monitoring, vigilance and further action remains, sometimes for generations.

For healthy children, reading is just what the doctor ordered

I t is the simplest, cheapest, most enjoyable way to give children a healthy start in life: read to them. Read aloud to your children and grandchildren. Read and sing and talk to them every day. Read to them until they can read for themselves. Then read together. And read to them some more until they start school, then encourage them to read even more. For optimal neurological development—nutrition for the brain, if you will—reading is just what the doctor ordered.

In fact, in a 2014 policy statement, the American Academy of Pediatrics took a strong stand on the importance of literacy to good health. The AAP, which represents sixty-two thousand US pediatricians, says physicians should prescribe "reading together as a daily fun family activity" every time a child has a doctor's visit and, for low-income children, provide age-appropriate books. To do so, they have teamed up with two wonderful organizations, Reach Out and Read and the Clinton Foundation's Too Small to Fail program, as well as the children's book publisher Scholastic. The new policy is getting a lot of attention in the United States, and rightfully so. Being illiterate, innumerate or uneducated almost always condemns one to poverty and poor health.

But let's not forgot that the Canadian Paediatric Society has had a similar position since way back in 2002—one it updated and made more forceful in 2011. While the CPS campaign has been much more low-key—unfortunately, they don't have the same clout and friends in high places as the AAP—its recommendations are even more sweeping. They say that waiting rooms should be chock full of books, that children should be handed books during visits because they are comforting, and in addition to kids being prescribed reading, they should be prescribed library cards and parents in need should be steered to literacy programs. Libraries provide an environment where learning can thrive and where there are no financial barriers.

The CPS statement also provides some chilling data on the "crisis of low literacy" in Canada. To wit:

- Forty-two percent of Canadians sixteen to sixty-five years of age do not have the minimum literacy skills for coping with everyday life and work in a knowledge-based economy.
- Low literacy skills are found among 80 percent of prison inmates, 60 percent of immigrants (compared with 37 percent of native-born Canadians) and 18 percent to 38 percent of youth, depending on the region of the country.
- Five percent to 15 percent of schoolchildren have reading delays, and most kids who have not mastered reading by the end of Grade 3 will never catch up.
- People with low literacy skills are twice as likely to be unemployed.
- Fifty percent of adults with low literacy levels live below the poverty line.
- Literacy problems cost Canada $10 billion a year.

"Not only is promoting literacy good medicine, it also makes economic sense," concludes the CPS.

Yet illiteracy, innumeracy and lack of education are, at their root, pediatric problems. A much-cited 2003 study by researchers at Kansas State University showed that, by age four, children of well-to-do professionals hear about thirty million more words than children of parents on social assistance, a gap they dubbed an "early catastrophe." This exposure to vocabulary—through reading, singing and talking—gives them a distinct advantage in school and carries through to school performance in later grades and, ultimately, to better education opportunities and higher-paying jobs. The statement from US pediatricians says that encouraging reading from an early age should help close the gaps between income and racial groups.

While reading to kids may seem like a no-brainer, in reality only about half of children are read to daily, and the principal reason given is there simply isn't enough time, especially with overworked parents and overprogrammed kids. With the proliferation of tablets and smartphones, the book may seem like an anachronism, but even if swiping replaces page-turning, reading aloud remains important. It not only stimulates neurons and builds vocabulary, but forges bonds between parents (or grandparents) and children.

Literacy is the foundation of a good education, and educational achievement is a good predictor of income. That trinity—literacy, education, income—is a powerful determinant of health. In fact, life expectancy, and health more generally, correlates pretty closely with education and income. Low literacy is an issue that health practitioners—beginning with pediatricians—cannot afford to ignore. A health system worthy of its name needs to promote literacy because it is a virtual prerequisite to good health.

Of course, your babies don't need to know all this. They just have to lie back and enjoy the bedtime stories, oblivious to the fact that the soothing words will provide more comfort and joy and good health than they can imagine.

The vaccine–autism debate should end now

Vaccines do not cause autism. The science proving this point has been quite clear for a number of years. But in February of 2009, the scientific evidence was given an important legal booster shot. Judges at the United States "vaccine court" ruled on three test cases in which it was claimed that the standard childhood vaccine for measles, mumps and rubella (MMR) caused autism, and they were unequivocal in their findings.

One judge, George Hastings (known by the title special master), said a thorough, dispassionate review of the evidence demonstrated that the vaccine–autism theory was "very wrong." He said parents who adhere to this theory "have been misled by physicians who are guilty ... of gross medical misjudgment." Special master Denise Vowell, who heard a case alleging that a mercury-based preservative called thimerosal can trigger autism, said that while the evidence is incredibly complex, the experts arguing that no link exists between autism and vaccines "were far more qualified, better supported by the weight of scientific research and authority, and simply more persuasive on nearly every point in contention." (Thimerosal was once used in childhood vaccines, but is no longer.) Special master Patricia Campbell-Smith, who heard the third test case, said that while one cannot help but be "moved as a person and as a parent" by the tragic stories of children with autism, there is simply no credible scientific evidence demonstrating a vaccine–autism link.

The judges considered five thousand pages of testimony from experts and 939 scientific articles and independently reached the same conclusion. The rulings from the "vaccine court"—which was set up as part of a US program to compensate people who suffer from occasional side effects of vaccines (Canada, with the exception of Quebec, does not have a compensation program for those harmed by vaccines)—effectively put an end to the cases of about forty-eight hundred families claiming their children's autism was caused by the MMR vaccine.

Unfortunately, the vaccine court is unlikely to put an end to unsubstantiated claims about the MMR vaccine and childhood vaccines more generally. That's because a whole industry of hucksters has sprung up to promote alternatives to vaccines, and the vocal (and Web-savvy) minority of conspiracy theorists will see these thorough, thoughtful rulings as, well, just another part of the conspiracy by Big Pharma to poison kids for profit.

The vaccine–autism scare dates back almost two decades. In 1998, British gastroenterologist Andrew Wakefield and colleagues published a now-infamous article in *The Lancet* medical journal that suggested a jab of MMR could trigger bowel conditions in children that led to autism. The study of twelve children caused a furor, but the findings have never been reproduced or substantiated. A number of Wakefield's co-authors have retracted parts of the paper and others are facing professional misconduct charges.

The damage has been incredible. In Britain, the number of children getting the MMR vaccine fell from 92 percent in 1996 to less than 80 percent in 2004, largely because of autism fears. The result was a resurgence of childhood illnesses such as measles and mumps. In Canada, the impact was lesser—with MMR vaccination rates dipping from 93 percent to 89 percent—but the vaccine–autism claims have fuelled an international anti-vaccine movement. It is a movement that relies on half-truths to peddle "alternatives" such as megadoses of vitamins, homeopathic medicines and sham autism treatments.

Yet this movement has flourished because public-health officials have been incredibly inept at promoting the benefits of vaccination and even worse at answering parents' legitimate concerns. The reality is that vaccines, and childhood vaccines in particular, are one of the greatest medical advances in the history of humanity. The virtual elimination of once-common conditions such as measles, mumps and diphtheria through childhood immunization programs has prevented thousands of deaths and untold suffering. In a way, vaccination programs have been a victim of their own success. Polio and smallpox are all but eradicated, and so uncommon now are diseases such as measles that the public has lost sight of the devastation they wrought.

The reality, too, is that all drugs have side effects and vaccines are no exception. Childhood vaccines—and Canadian kids now routinely get shots to protect them from fifteen illnesses—require bothersome needle sticks and they can cause fever and irritation. In rare instances, vaccines can cause shock, brain inflammation and death, particularly in children with allergies or compromised immune systems. But the risk needs to be kept in perspective: of the 400,000 children born in Canada each year—virtually all of whom are vaccinated—about five will have severe reactions. That makes vaccines many times safer than over-the-counter medications such as Aspirin and Tylenol.

The ultimate tragic irony in all this is that the MMR vaccine is probably the safest of all. Since the 1970s, more than half a billion doses of MMR have been administered around the world, and international research has concluded that there have been no deaths and no permanent damage caused by the vaccine. Parents should have these reassuring facts in plain language from health care professionals and public-health programs, not be dependent on massive court rulings or, worse yet, the alarmist dreck on the Web.

Canada should think inside the box on healthy babies

On June 4, 2013, the BBC News Magazine ran an astonishing story titled, "Why Finnish babies sleep in cardboard boxes." It was the tale of the "maternity package," a simple cardboard box loaded with goodies that every expectant mother receives in Finland. The gift from the state contains clothes, a snowsuit, bath products, cloth diapers, books, bedding and a mattress. Traditionally, newborns in the Nordic country spend many of their first naps and sleeps in that cardboard box, a practice related in the catchy headline.

While the contents of the box are significant and useful, even more important is the symbolism. The cardboard box says, "Every child matters. Every family matters." That philosophy is the cornerstone of Finnish public policy. It is not the box per se, but a wide range of child-centred and family-friendly social policies giving Finland argu-ably the healthiest children in the world. It is a philosophy that also helps explain why Finland has the world's happiest mothers, according to Save the Children.

Which invites the question, how does Canada compare? Well, to begin with, our moms come in at a mediocre twentieth place on the happiness ranking. More importantly, Finland has an infant mortality rate of 2.3 per thousand live births. Canada's rate is a shameful 5.7 per thousand—more than double. Why?

It begins with the box—or the message in the box. To collect the maternity package, Finnish moms-to-be must visit a maternity clinic. The contents, worth several hundred dollars, are an enticement to seek care. (Women can opt for a cash payment of 140 euros, but few do.) Practically, that means every pregnant woman gets care: not only medical interventions like ultrasound scans, but milk and fresh fruit. Prevention is the best way to reduce the number of low-birth-weight babies. The box contains a book on how to breastfeed, and every new Finnish mom gets a home visit from a lactation consultant. In Canada, our primary care is lacking and well-baby visits are a rarity. Until not too long ago, new moms were sent home with formula. In Finland, all new moms get nine months of maternity benefits—whether they work or not. Daycare is provided at no cost, and parents who choose to forgo daycare get a cash subsidy.

In Canada, maternity benefits flow from the employment-insurance program. Only if you pay in—meaning, essentially, you have a job with benefits—can you collect. The approach excludes students, many part-timers, the self-employed, those who are paid under the table, the unemployed and so on. The only province that has state-funded daycare is Quebec, and parents still pay $7 a day (if they can find a spot). Many parents pay $40 to $50 daily for child care, a usurious amount.

For a long time, Canada had a baby bonus. It started at $5 for each of "Johnny Canuck's offspring" after World War II and rose gradually until it was eliminated in the cost-cutting of the early 1990s. Today, Canada has a universal child-care benefit of $100 a month (taxable) and a child tax benefit for parents of children under six. Supplements are available for low-income parents and those with children with disabilities. These programs are paltry at best. They have helped reduce the breadth of poverty, but not its depths.

Countries like Finland simply do not allow children and families to wallow in poverty. It is socially and politically unacceptable. They recognize, implicitly and explicitly in public policy, that there is a cost to child-rearing for individuals and a benefit to society more broadly if children are raised healthy. So they facilitate parenting with a range of supports in health care, child care, education, housing and employment. It all begins with a cardboard box, a symbol of commitment.

In Canada, we don't have a family policy to speak of. We have a lot of rhetoric and very few concrete supports, financial or otherwise.

It's every mom for herself. We don't even provide a box of essentials, and that speaks volumes. If you don't get the building blocks right, then how do you produce a nation of healthy children?

———⊣⊢———

Children's pain gets short shrift

When children end up in hospital, we assume everything will be done to care for them, including minimizing pain. Unfortunately, that assumption is wrong. Two 2014 research papers serve as a grim reminder that pain is systematically undertreated in children.

One study, led by Kathryn Birnie of the Centre for Pediatric Pain Research at Dalhousie University in Halifax, found that fewer than half of hospitalized children have a pain-management plan. In other words, controlling pain is often an afterthought. The paper, published in the medical journal *Pain Research and Management*, also shows that even so-called low-intensity pain matters a lot to patients. A second paper, published in the *Canadian Journal of Emergency Medicine*, also shows wide variations in how children are treated for pain in the emergency room. The research team, led by Dr. Samina Ali of the department of pediatrics at the University of Alberta, found that the decision to give pain medication, or what strength is used, can be very different from one hospital to the next, regardless of the ailment or procedure.

Both papers show that younger children tend to get especially short shrift. "Most people don't take pain seriously," said Dr. Christine Chambers, a Dalhousie University professor who is also the Canada Research Chair in Pain and Child Health. She said Canadian health professionals aren't taught enough about it—veterinarians get five times as much education on pain management as physicians. And parents tend to mistakenly think either not much can be done or everything possible is being done to control their child's pain. They have to be demanding, which shouldn't be the case. It's not that doctors and nurses don't care. Pain relief just isn't seen as a priority when there are so many demands on their time.

Until the 1980s, babies, and premature infants in particular, received no pain relief at all, even when they underwent procedures like open-heart surgery. Instead of anesthetics to control pain, they were given paralytics to keep them from moving. The belief that babies don't feel pain was widespread, but nonsensical. Every parent knows they do. The notion that anesthetics were too dangerous for children has also been disproved. Practice changed dramatically when, in 1983, Dr. Kanwaljeet (Sunny) Anand, a pediatric pain specialist at Le Bonheur Children's Hospital in Memphis, Tennessee, published research showing that babies who did not get anesthetics during surgery suffered far more complications and were more likely to die than those who did get pain relief. Since then, our knowledge of pain has undergone a revolution. Yet some procedures, like circumcision outside of hospitals, can still take place without pain relief.

While anesthesia is now the norm during surgery, the research shows we still lag on controlling postsurgical pain. We're also more miss than hit on controlling chronic pain. At least children with cancer, who used to die excruciating deaths, now benefit from much better pain control. But the study of pain practices in the emergency room demonstrates that we still don't do near enough to relieve procedural and "routine" pain, such as that from vaccination needles and routine dental procedures. (Children now get about twenty shots before they're five, and often a few cavities filled.) When these young ones get poked and prodded—heel pricks, IV lines, catheters, blood tests, vaccines—everything should be done to minimize their pain, which can be considerable and traumatizing.

We have a wealth of knowledge of what works, including topical analgesics (rubbing a bit of cream on a child's arm ahead of time can reduce needle pain), breastfeeding, distraction, sugar water, skin-to-skin contact and Tylenol, to name a few. "It doesn't have to hurt," is how a video produced by IWK Children's Hospital in Halifax puts it. And it shouldn't.

Pain is very subjective. But not taking it seriously is cruel and can have lasting impacts. Suffering does not make kids tougher—on the contrary, it leaves psychological scars. Pain during childhood interventions, even routine vaccinations and dental freezing, can make people less likely to seek medical and dental care when they get older. And the sad fact is that, in Canada today, Chambers reminds us, "your dog could get better pain care than your child." That's not right. We need to heed our children's cries.

Guilty verdict is correct
for meningitis death

D avid and Collet Stephan failed to seek medical care for their nine-teen-month-old son, Ezekiel, in a timely fashion, and he died. For that, they were found guilty of failing to provide the necessities of life, and rightly so. The parents' failings were egregious: their toddler became increasingly ill, to the point where he was lethargic and stiff as a board; they were told by a nurse that the boy was likely suffering from meningitis, a life-threatening condition; they were urged by a naturopath to bring the child to a doctor, but they did not, opting instead for naturopathic "treatments" such as an Echinacea tincture. They didn't call 911 until Ezekiel stopped breathing and, by the time he was airlifted to hospital, it was too late to save him. Despite the conviction, they remained unrepentant, painting themselves as per-secuted and warning that the parenting police are out to get us all.

Hardly. The message in the conviction is consistent with what our laws and courts have said over decades in cases with similar philo-sophical underpinnings—parents who refuse blood transfusion, vac-cination, cancer treatment and other demonstrably beneficial medical treatments for their children in favour of prayer or other nonsense. As an adult, you can have beliefs, religious or otherwise, and you can raise your children according to those beliefs, no matter how wacky, but that does not obviate the obligation to provide the necessities of life. When a child's health and well-being are compromised, the rules change, because a guardian has responsibilities as well as rights. Put another way, children cannot give consent to the denial of treatment, so they are entitled to the accepted standard of care. In Ezekiel's case, he should have been treated with intravenous fluids, pain relief and antibiotics; what he got instead was chili-pepper smoothies and fluids from an eye-dropper. And that is criminal. (And to those who wonder whether conventional medicine could have saved the boy, the answer is: we'll never know. The parents' failure was not giving him a fighting chance.)

This case raises many difficult questions for regulators and policy-makers. Is naturopathy—a belief system that has no scientific basis—a legitimate health profession? After all, in Alberta and a number of other provinces, it is recognized as such, allowing naturopaths to self-regulate. Should Health Canada give legitimacy to the naturopathic and homeopathic concoctions such as those used on Ezekiel by approving and regulating "natural health products"? Again, there is no scientific evidence of their benefit. But the most important question of all is, why have Canadians embraced so-called complementary and alternative treatments so broadly and enthusiastically?

Much of what is espoused—take care of yourself, be attuned to your body, think about where your food comes from, and so on—is quite sensible and healthy. But a lot of pseudoscientific nonsense is also out there, from homeopathy (with its ridiculous core belief that diluting medicine in water makes it stronger) to the rejection of vaccines as poison—much of it promoted by "alternative" practitioners such as naturopaths and chiropractors and high-profile crackpots like Dr. Joseph Mercola—that too many people embrace uncritically. What people seem to be yearning for is some control over their health, and some hands-on care, things that are all-too-often unavailable in the rushed, paternalistic mainstream health system. They also are skeptical—and not entirely without reason—of some of the machinations of pharmaceutical companies.

Pseudoscience is comforting: it's easy to embrace, promising magic and definitive answers, not all messy and rife with unanswered questions like real science. Add to this a lot of flowery language about "natural," "holistic" and "drug-free" treatments, and a dash of scientific illiteracy, and you have a potent cocktail that can occasionally have horrible consequences.

Beyond the death of Ezekiel, however, the real tragedy is that a lot of David and Collet Stephans are out there—parents who are well-meaning but are nonetheless harming their children. The answer is not to prosecute and jail them all; it is to educate them, and to above all else encourage them to be at least as doubtful and skeptical about "alternative" treatments as they are mainstream ones.

In this case, nobody argued that the parents harmed their child deliberately but, as the prosecutor said at the end of the trial, "Sometimes love just isn't enough." Sometimes—no, all the time—making the right choices to ensure a child's well-being has to supersede all other considerations. When you fail to do so, like Ezekiel's parents, you have to take your medicine.

CHAPTER 8

Reproductive/ Women's Health

Dr. Henry Morgentaler's lasting
mark on health care

Say what you will about Dr. Henry Morgentaler—and there are few things, good, bad and despicably ugly, that have not been said about him—but he forever changed the face of health care in Canada. His crusade to legalize abortion and to make safe medical abortions available across the country has greatly benefited the health of Canadian women. It has made the delivery of health care more just—and by extension, our society.

In 1967, Morgentaler appeared before a House of Commons committee and delivered a tongue-lashing to politicians, along with an unvarnished account of the horrors of backstreet abortions using knitting needles and Drano injections. The next year, he performed his first abortion, then, in 1969, openly defied the law by opening a private abortion clinic. In 1970, the pro-choice doctor was arrested and acquitted. The acquittal was later overturned, and he served ten months of an eighteen-month prison before being released. The legal battles multiplied until the issue made its way to the highest court—twice.

In 1975, Morgentaler's bid to quash the restrictions on abortion failed in the Supreme Court of Canada. But in 1987—after the Canadian Charter of Rights and Freedoms became law—he tried again. His lawyer argued that denying women timely access to abortion violated the Constitution—specifically Section 7 of the Charter, which guarantees "life, liberty, and security of the person." The Supreme Court agreed and, on January 28, 1988, abortion was decriminalized. Since then, there has been no federal law.

The fact that Canada has gone three decades without an abortion law reminds us that Canadian society shows a pretty broad consensus that, while no one revels in having an abortion, the choice needs to be there and that deeply personal choice ultimately rests with every woman. The consensus, too, is that when abortions are performed—and there are about 105,000 a year in Canada—they should be done safely and covered by medicare, like other medically necessary procedures.

Yet while abortion is safe, legal and publicly funded in Canada, there are still many practical hurdles for a woman seeking to terminate a pregnancy. Many provinces continue to flout the letter and the spirit of the Morgentaler ruling. Nationwide, only about one in five hospitals performs abortions—at least on paper. But even those that do offer the service impose arbitrary gestation limits and have lengthy wait-lists. Many women still have to travel out of province for the procedure, and some provinces still refuse to pay for abortions in private clinics. Not to mention that women who wish to have an abortion, and the doctors who perform abortions, still must endure harassment and abuse from the "pro-life" zealots who stake out clinics. The Morgentaler Clinic in Toronto was actually firebombed in 1992, and Morgentaler pointedly refused to don a bulletproof vest in public as police urged him to do because, ironically, he was the subject of so many death threats.

Besides health care, Morgentaler also left an indelible mark on Canadian law. Since 1998, more than four hundred court rulings have made reference to the Morgentaler decision on issues ranging from the limits of free speech to the access to private health care. One of the ironies of the decision was that, by ensuring timely access to a basic service, the court paved the way for a system of private abortion clinics. The reality is that the private clinics should never have been required. The private clinics, operated by Morgentaler and others, became necessary only because governments failed to carry out their constitutional responsibilities.

Morgentaler was also a polarizing political figure. In 2008, after years of lobbying and much criticism of the advisory committee, he was invested into the Order of Canada. At the time, I wrote that it was unconscionable that such a towering figure should be overlooked so long for the country's highest honour: "Traditional honours, be they honorary degrees or the Order of Canada, should not be reserved for marshmallows, nor for antiseptic public figures. They should—and must—recognize that great achievements often result from monumental battles, and that those who defend fundamental rights rarely win popularity contests."

When Morgentaler died on May 29, 2013, a deafening silence followed from the country's elite rather than the usual outpouring of praise and remembrance for public figures. The title of Catherine Dunphy's definitive biography, *Morgentaler: A Difficult Hero*, says it all. He was peevish, arrogant and authoritarian. He inspired more exasperation than love, even among his most committed allies. But he nevertheless made Canada a place where most women can have safe, legal and affordable access to abortion when they need it. A place where—unlike much of the world—women don't have to resort to using coat hangers in back alleys to assert their reproductive rights.

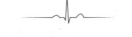

It's not just about the pill anymore

In 2016, the Planned Parenthood Federation of America turned one hundred years old. It reached its peak during the sexual revolution, and it flourished because of desperate need. Just as the pill arrived on the scene, a growing number of women were entering the workforce and wanted to delay childbearing to pursue careers. The radical notion that women should have some say over how many children to have, and when, also took hold.

Yet there was fearsome resistance from traditionalists, church leaders and lawmakers. Until 1969, prescribing contraceptives was illegal in Canada. So, too, was abortion. But demand for both was soaring. A small group of brave, outspoken women filled the gap, pioneers of the family-planning movement, as it was then called. Planned Parenthood was at the forefront. Volunteers set up small clinics offering practical, non-judgmental advice, as they do to this day. They steered women to sympathetic doctors (at the time, the pill could be prescribed for menstrual problems, a loophole that was widely exploited) and offered sage counsel on sexual and reproductive issues.

Today, there are more than ten million prescriptions filled annually for contraceptive products in Canada, and sales exceed $300 million (excluding over-the-counter products such as condoms). While use of birth control pills is steadily declining, the popularity of intrauterine devices (IUDs) and fertility tracking apps is growing. Yet groups like the former Planned Parenthood Federation of Canada (the Canadian Federation for Sexual Health, an umbrella group with twenty-three affiliates and ties to like-minded groups around the world) are needed more than ever. Abortion has been decriminalized but access remains spotty and unequal, as the anti-choice movement continues its rear-guard action. A dizzying array of contraceptive options is available, but deciding on one is difficult. Avoiding pregnancy is now only one part of the equation, with the advent of HIV-AIDS and the multitude of other sexually transmitted infections.

Because schools have, by and large, abdicated their responsibilities, sex education of young people remains abysmal. They get their (mis) education from peers and from hypersexualized images in the media, in movies and online. Hypocritically, we demand that teenagers and young adults be responsible, but we fail to give them the tools to act responsibly. For younger generations like millennials, family planning now often involves not just birth control but struggles with all manner of technology to enhance fertility. And the Viagra generation—the baby boomers who grew up liberated but not particularly informed about sex—are looking for guidance as they shift from worrying about pregnancy to concerns about flagging libidos and navigating sex after cancer. Multiculturalism, too, poses unique challenges, as women and men seek reproductive and sexual education that is culturally relevant, and in a language they can understand.

For all these reasons and more, Planned Parenthood changed a lot over the years, including changing its name to the Canadian

Federation for Sexual Health and then to Action Canada for Sexual Health and Rights. The move was appropriate and overdue. The more than 300,000 people who go to ACSHR for help each year are rarely looking for family-planning advice per se. The majority of the clientele are young women—teenaged and college age—who are sexually active or considering being so. Increasingly, young men with the same insecurities are going, too. In an era of "friends with benefits," "lesbians until graduation," blurring gender lines, ecstasy-fuelled raves, the morning-after pill, menstrual suppression, born-again virgins, unlimited porn on the Web, and seemingly higher rates of oral and anal sex among high schoolers, the counselling sessions of today in no way resemble those of a half century ago. Young people today have a lot more information about sex, but they don't necessarily have more knowledge or wisdom. So the curiosity and questions remain.

Today's youth need a champion of reproductive and sexual health as much as ever. In its mission statement, the ACSHR group says it is trying to create a "global society that celebrates healthy sexuality, its diversity of expression and reproductive choice as fundamental human rights for individuals throughout life." Instead of bemoaning the fact that teenagers are—shock, horror!—having sex, instead of obsessing about what carnal acts are à la mode (oral sex is slightly more popular than intercourse), we should be ensuring that our children grow up knowing that healthy sexuality is an integral part of a healthy life. Young people today—and older people, for that matter—don't need to hear lectures on the mechanics of sex or see more hackneyed sex-ed films. We need to celebrate, not repress, sexuality.

For that to happen, we need a forum for honest discussion about choices, the need for respect and the self-imposed limits that are an integral part of healthy sexuality at any age. Schools are not providing that forum. Many parents are too squeamish and are not providing that opportunity at home. So do your children and grand-children a favour and slip them the number (or better yet, the URL, www.sexualhealthandrights.ca/) for Action Canada. You'll know their sexual health is in good hands.

Stillbirths: Motherhood's silent scourge

W hen Christine Jonas-Simpson's son Ethan was born, there was an eerie quiet in the delivery room, and then a piercing wail. "The only cry I heard was my own," she said sombrely. Ethan was dead, "born still" in the language of grieving parents; "stillborn" in the medical vernacular. The umbilical cord was constricted, essentially suffocating the baby in the womb, a condition impossible to detect with an ultrasound.

Jonas-Simpson, who was almost thirty-eight weeks pregnant, knew her son was dead before she went into labour. When he was born, she held Ethan in her arms, stroking his shock of curly red hair. So did her husband. The nurses were wonderfully supportive, even explaining to Ethan's young siblings how his air tube was broken, something that could happen to an astronaut. The family was able to mourn on their terms. (Jonas-Simpson, a professor of nursing at York University, published a children's book, *Ethan's Butterflies*, and produced a series of research papers and documentaries on stillbirth, the latest of which, *Enduring Love: Transforming Loss*, premiered in Toronto on May 15, 2011.)

Unlike Ethan, most babies born still are quickly "disposed of" without being held, named or given a funeral. In much of the world, reproduction is central to a woman's purpose, so there is profound stigma, and no small measure of blame falls on the mother when childbirth fails to produce a living child. Data published in 2015 show that more than 2.6 million stillbirths occur worldwide each year. The deaths remain largely uncounted, the mothers unsupported and preventive measures understudied. It is an epidemic—one that claims more lives each year than HIV-AIDS and malaria combined—that quietly unfolds far from the public eye.

In April 2011, *The Lancet* published a series of articles that aimed to shatter the silence by examining the staggering toll of stillbirth—emotional, physical and economic—and proposing practical solutions.

A stillbirth, as defined by the World Health Organization, is one in which a baby dies after reaching at least twenty-eight weeks gestation and weighing at least one thousand grams. In a country like Canada with advanced medical care, it is twenty-two weeks at five hundred grams. (Loss of a fetus before that time is considered a miscarriage or, if the pregnancy is terminated, an abortion.)

There is a common belief that babies who die in utero were never meant to live. Stillbirths have been seen as a form of natural selection, bad luck, the result of witchcraft—lame seventeenth-century explanations for a lingering twenty-first-century scourge. The other myth is that most stillbirths occur early in the pregnancy. In fact, the opposite is true: the longer the gestation, the higher the risk.

Yet the vast majority of stillbirths are preventable. In wealthy countries like Canada, where high-tech obstetrics are the norm, stillbirths are linked to smoking, obesity, advanced maternal age and abnormalities in the placenta and umbilical cord. Worldwide, fewer than 5 percent are due to congenital abnormalities like anencephaly (lack of a brain stem), and many of those conditions are caused by lack of essential nutrients like folic acid. The 1.4 million babies who die antepartum (before delivery) each year tend to succumb because their mothers have preventable or treatable conditions like syphilis, malaria, diabetes or hypertension. The 1.2 million babies who die intrapartum (during delivery) do so because they lack access to even the most basic obstetrical care, such as a midwife who can assist with a breech birth. These deaths are dismissively listed as resulting from "complications."

But the real complications are poverty and lack of access to basic health-care services for women. Bear in mind that of the 131 million births worldwide annually, at least 60 million women deliver alone, invariably those who live in the most squalid conditions. Needless to say, the great majority of stillbirths occur in the developing world. Five countries—India, Pakistan, Nigeria, China and Bangladesh—account for more than half. China, it should be noted, has dramatically reduced its rate of stillbirths in recent years. Worldwide, rates range from two per one thousand births in Finland to forty per one thousand in Nigeria. Canada's rate is 3.3 per one thousand births, but the rate of stillbirths is three times higher in Inuit and First Nations communities than in the general population. Stated bluntly, stillbirth is inversely correlated with wealth; the problem exists largely where there is rampant poverty, no education and poor housing, like all conditions that stalk mothers and children. Each year, more than 400,000 women die in childbirth and about three million babies die. Stillbirth is the unspoken part of the puzzle.

In recent years, determined and fairly successful efforts have been made to prevent mothers from dying while birthing and to protect babies from the infectious diseases, malnutrition and traumatic injuries that kill, thanks largely to investment in the Millennium Development Goals. (In 2000, 189 countries agreed to embrace the MDGs—eight goals with measurable targets and clear deadlines for improving the lives of the world's poorest people.) But reducing stillbirths is, inexplicably, not one of the millennium goals. The problem has largely been ignored by the global public-health community. Instead of a plan, there is fatalism.

In its articles, *The Lancet* not only exposes the problem but proposes solutions that include investment in family planning, obstetric care, bed nets to protect against malaria and screening for syphilis. These measures would, according to the published calculations, reduce stillbirths by 45 percent, meaning 1.1 million fewer deaths a year.

In recent years, the focus has been on safe motherhood and on improved child survival after live birth. It is now time to put some effort into ensuring that more children are born alive. These lives that will never be lived—a source of incalculable heartbreak—cry out for attention.

INTERVENTION	PREVENTED STILLBIRTHS
Emergency obstetric care	696,000
Syphilis detection and treatment	136,000
Management of fetal growth restriction	107,000
Managing high blood pressure during pregnancy	57,000
Induction for mothers with more than 41 weeks gestation	52,000
Malaria prevention, including bed nets and drugs	35,000
Folic acid fortification before conception	27,000
Managing diabetes in pregnancy	24,000

Source: *The Lancet*, 2011

It's time to stop treating
pregnancy like a disease

The number-one reason for hospitalization in Canada is childbirth. The most commonly performed surgery in this country is the Caesarean section. Those facts should give us all a case of morning sickness. And they should prompt a lot of hard questions. Is pregnancy a disease? Is a hospital really the best place to give birth? Are women ending up there by choice or by default? Is surgery actually required to deliver one in every five babies?

In 2015–16, there were 392,902 live births in Canada, according to Statistics Canada; in 2014–15, there were 366,703 births in hospitals, according to the Canadian Institute for Health Information (CIHI). The balance were home births or babies born in birthing centres not located in a hospital. (Also, StatCan counts actual babies; for CIHI, multiple births—twins and up—count as a single birth.) All that is to say that roughly 98 percent of Canadian babies are born in hospitals. And virtually every baby in this country is still delivered under the supervision of a physician—either a specialist obstetrician-gynecologist or a general practitioner. Fewer than 5 percent of births involve a midwife.

Let's face it—most births are uncomplicated. That doesn't mean easy—it means not requiring medical intervention. Where and how you give birth matters. If you put a perfectly healthy pregnant woman in a hospital, she becomes a patient—someone to be monitored, sedated, drugged, "assisted," operated on and so on. When someone is placed in an institutional setting, often a cascade of dubious and not always useful interventions occurs: shaving of pubic hair, fetal monitoring, IV drips, inducement, epidurals, forceps, episiotomy and, often, a Caesarean section. (Again, this is not to suggest that epidurals are unnecessary, and 58 percent of women opt for one during delivery, but pain relief can be done outside the hospital, too.)

In 2014 in Canada, 100,843 C-sections were performed—27.5 percent of births. Does anyone seriously believe that level is justified? The World Health Organization suggests that the optimal rate is somewhere between 5 and 15 percent. Too many C-sections are done for the sake of convenience (of the physician, rarely the patient) and out of fear. For example, women over thirty-five are twice as likely to have a C-section as those under thirty-five; low-income patients are also far more likely to go under the knife. Don't buy the "too posh to push" nonsense. Yes, an increasing number of women are "choosing" a Caesarean, but when you medicalize pregnancy and labour and don't offer reasonable alternatives, you create uncertainty and fear. And just as troubling as the high rate of C-sections overall is the wide variability in rates around the country, ranging from 15 percent in Quebec to 37 percent in New Brunswick. (The C-section rate in Nunavut is only 10 percent, but high-risk pregnancies are handled out of territory so it's not a fair comparison.)

Yes, surgery can be lifesaving. But too much surgery is harmful. Physicians should be handling the complex, high-risk cases—women with conditions such as obesity and heart disease that compromise the pregnancy, mothers over thirty-five (though the risks to "older" women are debatable) and so on. Most births can and should be handled by midwives, preferably in a home-like setting such as a birthing centre. This is not an attempt to romanticize "natural" childbirth or a call to return to the "good old days"—because they weren't so good. Until the last century, babies were born at home with little support and many tragic complications for moms and babies alike. Maternal mortality fell precipitously in the twentieth century, but only a small portion of those improvements happened because of obstetrical interventions.

Today, we have a much higher standard of living (hence healthier mothers), we have contraception and emancipation (so the days of seventeen children are mercifully behind us) and, most of all, we have better infection control, including vaccination and antiseptic environments. The greatest risks to our foremothers were infectious diseases and excessive bleeding. Those are still the biggest risks today, but they are manageable risks. In a bid to entirely remove risk (which is not possible), we have made pregnancy and birth unnecessarily tedious and costly and created new risks to boot.

To make our health system patient-centred, efficient and cost-effective, the aim should be to deliver appropriate care in the right place at the right time with the right health professional. Profound cultural change is required—and what better place to start than by tackling the leading cause of hospitalization and in-patient surgery? Pregnancy and birthing are part of a normal physiological process that should be celebrated. Bringing a child into the world should be beautiful and memorable, messy and magical. Why have we reduced it to a series of billable acts where moms-to-be are institutionalized and the process is unnecessarily medicalized? Mothers and their babies deserve better.

Sexist rules deny women true
reproductive choice

When the abortion pill was finally approved by Health Canada in July 2015—twenty-seven years after it came on the market in France—the news was greeted with a mixture of relief and elation. But after Health Canada released the regulatory conditions for the drug's use, there was consternation anew. The additional delays meant it was not on pharmacy shelves until January 2017.

The principal benefit of the drug, sold under the brand name Mifegymiso, is convenience. To induce an abortion, you take medication rather than undergo surgery. Abortion is legal in Canada, but access to surgery remains inadequate, which is why access to the abortion pill is essential. This is particularly true outside big cities, and for women who face religious and cultural barriers to terminating a pregnancy. But the regulatory hurdles for getting the drug are numerous, onerous and, for the most part, unjustified.

Mifegymiso consists of two drugs. Mifepristone works by blocking the hormone progesterone; without it, the lining of the uterus breaks down and the pregnancy cannot continue. The second drug, misoprostol, taken twenty-four to forty-eight hours later, causes the uterus to empty, similar to a miscarriage. (The abortion pill is not to be confused with the morning-after pill, levonorgestrel, commonly known as Plan B, which prevents a fertilized egg from latching on to the uterus and thus prevents pregnancy.)

Under the new rules, the drug must be prescribed and dispensed by doctors, which means they have to keep it in stock in their office. It is also obligatory for physicians to take an online course before they are allowed to prescribe. Before women can be prescribed the abortion pill, they must undergo an ultrasound and, most troubling of all, doctors can oblige a woman to take the drug under supervision, in their office. No doubt these measures are well-intentioned, to ensure safety, but they are also patronizing and sexist. One would be hard-pressed to identify any other drug that comes with such sweeping preconditions to access. Even the chemotherapy drug methotrexate, which is currently used off-label to induce abortion, has no such restrictions. The abortion pill has been used for almost three decades and is safer than many drugs on the market—including Viagra, the erectile-dysfunction drug for men.

In Canada, Mifegymiso is approved for use up to forty-nine days after conception. An ultrasound can be used to determine the age of the fetus. However, timing of conception can also be accurately measured without an ultrasound. The other reason for an ultrasound is to detect an ectopic pregnancy (where the embryo grows outside the uterus) or molar pregnancy (where the placenta develops into a mass of cysts). These conditions are rare and, again, can often be detected by other means. Ultrasound is not a bad idea, but it should not be mandatory, especially if it impedes access or results in additional cost. (Mifegymiso, distributed in Canada by Celopharma Inc., costs about $300, roughly the same as a surgical abortion.)

Doctor-dispensed drugs are a rarity. This condition is usually imposed to ensure that a drug is taken and not trafficked on the streets—such as methadone. There is no evidence women who want to terminate a pregnancy would try to sell Mifegymiso on the black market. There is no reason it cannot be dispensed by pharmacists, like virtually every other prescription drug, nor any reason it cannot be prescribed by nurse practitioners or midwives, as it is in many countries.

The most worrisome rule of all is the suggestion that the abortion pill must be taken in the presence of a physician. It's not always easy to get a timely appointment with a doctor in Canada. And why would a woman be forced to sit in a doctor's office while she has the equivalent of a miscarriage? We don't make women sit in doctors' offices during their miscarriages or periods, and we shouldn't oblige them to do so during medical abortions either. But they should be counselled to seek immediate emergency medical help if they see signs of infection and follow up to ensure the treatment worked (it does not work in about 2 percent of cases).

Like all drugs, Mifegymiso has possible side effects, such as allergic reaction and severe bleeding. The most dangerous potential side effects are bacterial infection and sepsis (blood poisoning)—but these symptoms are not immediate and need to be treated in a hospital. The risk is not from the pill per se, but from bleeding, and the risks are similar to surgical abortion, miscarriage, menstruation and childbirth, which all create conditions for infection.

Safety is important, but so is access. And right now the balance is tipped the wrong way, denying Canadian women true reproductive choice. Both surgical and drug-induced abortions are safe and effective procedures. Their availability should be based on science—not politics, religious beliefs, moral judgments or prudishness. About 105,000 Canadian women undergo abortions each year. In exercising choice, they should also have choices.

Heart disease isn't just for men, after all

"Men explode, but women erode." That's how Carolyn Thomas, who blogs under the moniker My Heart Sisters, sums up how heart attacks can differ between men and women. In men, arterial plaque breaks off, causing a clot and crushing chest pain—a Hollywood-style, chest-clutching heart attack. In women, plaque tends to erode, gradually blocking the artery, so they suffer fatigue and pain around the shoulders, back and arm.

But even when women present with classic heart attack symptoms—chest pain, nausea, sweating and pain radiating down the left arm—like Thomas did in May 2008—they are often misdiagnosed. Women's heart attacks are misdiagnosed between 26 and 54 percent of the time, according to the published research. Thomas was told she had acid reflux and sent home, but not before apologizing to the emergency room doctor for being a bother. Days later, she suffered a classic "widowmaker"—99 percent arterial blockage—and nearly died. (Maybe it should be called in a "widower-maker" in women?)

She has since dedicated herself to raising awareness that cardiovascular disease is not strictly a man's disease and that there are significant gender differences in how heart disease occurs and should be treated.

In 2012, 66,178 Canadians died of cardiovascular disease—33,196 women and 32,982 men. That's more women than men, in case you didn't notice. In fact, cardiovascular disease is the leading cause of death, disability and hospitalization for women over the age of thirty-five. Yet the public and even health-care practitioners often labour under the belief that heart disease is a man's disease and cancer is a woman's disease. As Dr. Noel Bairey Merz, director of the Barbra Streisand Women's Heart Health Center at Cedars-Sinai Heart Institute in Los Angeles, said in a 2011 TED Talk: "Breast cancer ... kills women, but heart disease kills a whole bunch more."

Recognition is also growing that cardiovascular disease needs to be treated differently in women. That's the motivation for the creation, in 2014, of the Canadian Women's Heart Health Centre—the first of its kind in Canada—at the University of Ottawa Heart Institute. "The landscape of women and heart disease has evolved greatly over the years, but efforts still need to be made in addressing the lack of public and professional awareness of women's coronary risk," said Dr. Michele Turek, the centre's medical adviser. "We must address this important challenge and correct misperceptions concerning the incidence, prevalence and significance of cardiovascular disease."

Biological differences between the sexes must be considered. For example, women develop cardiovascular disease, on average, seven to ten years later than men. They also have specific risks related to pregnancy: women who suffer pre-eclampsia or gestational diabetes have significantly higher risks of heart disease later in life. We know, too, that a woman's risk of heart attack or stroke soars after menopause—because blood pressure, cholesterol and diabetes rates all increase.

But most risk factors are common to women and men. The main reason women with heart disease have worse outcomes is not physically because of gender, but because prevention is lacking and treatment is delayed. That's why the centre in Ottawa is focused on prevention and providing strategies and resources. Because the issue is not on the radar for health providers or women themselves, there tends to be less prevention work done and significant differences in treatment—and not in a good way. Until a generation ago, cardiovascular research focused almost exclusively on men. And despite efforts to raise awareness, the treatment gap remains notable. Women get fewer angiograms, less surgery (either revascularization or bypass) and fewer stents. They are less likely to be prescribed daily ASA and ACE inhibitors for prevention, and less likely to get statins, beta blockers and ACE inhibitors as treatment. It wasn't until 2004 that the first gender-specific treatment guidelines for cardiovascular disease were published.

Given all this, it's not surprising that women have higher death rates—38 percent of women die within a year of having a heart attack, compared to 25 percent of men. And, while heart-related deaths are falling overall—due largely to the decrease in smoking rates—they are falling much more quickly for men than for women. In the past thirty-five years, cardiovascular mortality has dropped 17 percent in men, but just 2 percent in women. There is still a lot of catching up to be done, but it starts with awareness.

CHAPTER 9

Disability/ Inclusion

Everyone deserves the right
to reach for the sky

C hantal Petitclerc is the picture of good health. With twenty-one Olympic medals, she is one of the most outstanding athletes in Canadian history. No qualifying adjective is required. No asterisk appears beside her world records. The gold on the fourteen medals she collected in Olympic Games—from 1992, 1996, 2000, 2004 and 2008—is no less lustrous than medals belonging to racers who use form-fitted shoes instead of streamlined chairs. Yet when we speak of Petitclerc (who is now a Senator) and her stunning athletic and other accomplishments, the starting point is too often her disability, the fact that she uses a wheelchair.

The same is true of our attitude toward the other 3.8 million Canadians living with disabilities—physical, developmental and psychiatric (from StatCan's 2012 Canadian Survey on Disability). Individually or collectively, we too often slap "them" with the label *disabled*, and we do so dismissively. This condescending attitude was glaringly evident when Petitclerc was named co-winner of the prize as the country's top track-and-field athlete, rather than the outright winner. Athletics Canada was hammered, and rightly so, for that decision—which clearly implies that a disabled athlete, no matter how dominating, cannot compare with an able-bodied one.

But sport is not the only area where people with disabilities are treated unjustly. A patronizing approach also pervades public policy.

The health and social welfare systems tend to classify the full range of people with disabilities as needy—the factory worker who loses his legs in an industrial accident, the man with Down syndrome employed by the YMCA, the stockbroker with bipolar disorder, and the retired teacher blinded by macular degeneration—and relegates them to specific treatment and assistance programs.

While many treatment programs are excellent—though often in short supply—the "assistance" programs are often anything but. The greatest threat to the health of many people with disabilities is not their underlying medical condition, but poverty—income being one of the most powerful determinants of health. Even so, people with disabilities across all demographics are systematically marginalized. Children with disabilities are poorly integrated into the school system, which results in a lower level of education that translates into lower income later in life. Seniors, the age group where disability rates are highest, find themselves doubly isolated in a society built for speed and uniformity. Yet many people with disabilities do work—the majority of those of working age toil away like everyone else. Because most disabilities are invisible, they are hidden in plain sight. What we do know, however, is that most people with disabilities are not reaching their potential.

The 12 percent of the population living with disabilities want the same thing the other 88 percent want: a good life. As Al Etmanski, founder of the Planned Lifetime Advocacy Network, points out, a good life can be defined the same way for virtually everyone: "Friends and family, a place of your own, basic wealth, choice and—this is one that is too often forgotten—the ability to make a contribution to society." Etmanski says the key issue for people with disabilities is citizenship: if our commitment to rights and equality is real, then they need to be full citizens, meaning they have an equal opportunity to participate fully in all aspects of community life.

Equality, of course, does not mean sameness. But it does necessitate flexibility, accommodation and commitment. When Petitclerc was injured—her spine snapped by a barn door that fell on her—the community rallied: an elevator was installed at school and machinery was modified to work with hand controls. In gym class, she swam while others ran. Nice gestures all but, as full citizens, people with disabilities should not have to depend on generosity. Public buildings and workplaces should be accessible—not as an exception, but as a matter of course. So should parks, ski hills and beaches.

There will be grumbling that accessibility is costly, but in reality the changes that benefit the disability community benefit everyone: the mother pushing a baby carriage, the grandfather with fading eyesight and the child learning in an environment with his peers—all his peers. Access cannot be merely a token gesture. As Rick Hansen is fond of saying, "It's not enough to get in the theatre. You should be able to get on stage."

Which brings us to the real injustice that has befallen Petitclerc. Nobody in this country—perhaps in the world—better embodies the Olympic credo "faster, higher, stronger." So why was Petitclerc relegated to competing at the Paralympic Games, a week after the "real" Olympics? There is no place for such segregation in the Olympic movement, or in a just society. What Petitclerc has reminded us, through her deeds as well as her words, is that the yearning for belonging and meaning unites us all. The sooner she and other people with disabilities are afforded the full rights of citizenship, the richer we will all be.

—⎮⎮—

It's wrong to keep this
disabled girl as an "angel"

The history of treatment of people with physical, developmental and psychiatric disabilities is a bleak one, replete with systematic cases of abuse, both individual and collective. Because of their perceived shortcomings—mental retardation, twisted limbs, behaviours that violate social norms, being a burden on society—people with disabilities have been ostracized, lobotomized, sterilized, institutionalized, euthanized and even sent to the gas chambers. Sadly, in the twenty-first century, we continue to add new chapters to this age-old book of horrors.

Consider the case of Ashley X, a girl born in 1997 in Washington state who suffers from static encephalopathy (severe brain damage of unknown origin). She cannot walk, talk, roll over, sit up or speak. She essentially lies where she is placed, usually on a pillow, hence her moniker "pillow angel." In 2004, Ashley underwent a hysterectomy (removal of the uterus and ovaries), radical mastectomy (removal of the breast buds) and appendectomy, and she was infused with high doses of estrogen to fuse her bones together so they would stop growing. Ashley's parents, a middle-class, college-educated couple, requested these "growth attenuation" procedures to ensure she remains in a child's body for the remainder of her life.

Details of the case were published in the medical journal *Archives of Pediatric and Adolescent Medicine* in October 2006, and a few months later, the story vaulted into the mainstream press after the parents posted a defence of their action on a website (the updated site is http://pillowangel.org/). The response has been impassioned, to say the least. The couple, the girl's principal caregivers, argued (just as they did before the ethics board that approved the unusual medical experiment) that keeping Ashley small would facilitate her care and that depriving her of sexual characteristics would protect her from sexual abuse. The parents claimed that what they did to Ashley was not for their convenience but for the girl's comfort. They said the medical procedures were not cruel; rather, "what is grotesque is having a fully grown fertile woman endowed with the mind of a baby."

Without question, Ashley's parents love her. They care for her deeply and want the best for her. But what they did is wrong. It is beyond grotesque. The doctors involved in this butchery should be ashamed of their actions. They have violated one of the fundamental tenets of the ethical practice of medicine: never do deliberate harm to anyone for anyone else's interest. The surgeries and drugs have no direct benefit to the patient, and that makes them inappropriate. The sole purpose of growth attenuation is to keep Ashley portable and cute. And if cutting off the girl's breasts and amputating her uterus and ovaries is acceptable, why stop there? She is being tube-fed, so why not remove her teeth? Cutting off her arms and legs would certainly make her easier to dress. And she is incontinent, so why not replace her colon and bladder with colostomy and urostomy bags? A slippery slope? Indeed it is.

The parents say the only reason they have gone public is so other parents of "pillow angels" can learn of the treatment and follow suit. Since the story became public in 2004, at least six other children—four girls and two boys—have undergone the "Ashley Treatment." But what we are seeing here is a glaring manifestation of societal prejudice. Children with disabilities are seen as angelic and innocent; sexually functioning adults with disabilities, on the other hand, are viewed as disgusting and fearsome. Is it really true that using hoists and lifts to move people with severe disabilities is more dehumanizing than carrying them in your arms? Does the added burden of changing sanitary napkins in addition to continence pads really justify mutilation? Should not everyone, disabled or not, sexually mature or not, be protected from sexual abuse?

Her parents' last report in 2012 stated that Ashley takes the bus to school, where she spends a few hours every day. Like many parents of disabled children, that is the only respite her parents get from around-the-clock caregiving duties. Unquestionably, parents and their children of all ages with disabilities need more help, more support and more understanding. But in Ashley's case, the parents have corrected what did not need fixing. They have applied an invasive, ethically dubious medical solution to a pervasive social problem. The challenge of integrating people with disabilities into society, affording them the full rights of citizenship they are entitled to, is ever-present.

Due to advances in medical technology, an increasing number of children (and adults and seniors) are surviving with incredibly challenging conditions. Their care must be grounded in ethical decision-making, their rights protected as vigorously as those of everyone else in society. The way to deal with children with lifelong behavioural, physical and psychiatric problems is not to artificially maintain them in a permanent childlike body. Care, like people themselves, must evolve, grow and adapt. Children are not bonsai trees to be pruned and reshaped to suit the limitations or prejudices of their caregivers, or of society in general. Ashley, like every other child, is entitled to reach her full potential, no matter how inconvenient that may be to others.

Heartbreak city: Disabled kids

F ew things are more heartbreaking than a child with no friends. But being friendless is the norm for Canadian children with physical and developmental disabilities. A 2012 study, written by Dr. Anne Snowdon, a nurse and professor at the Odette School of Business at the University of Windsor in Ontario, shows that 53 percent of disabled kids have no friends. None.

Even those with friends have very limited interactions. Outside of formal settings such as the classroom, less than two hours a week spent with their peers is the norm; only 1 percent of children with disabilities spend an hour a day with friends. The problem is most serious for boys—who tend to have far more developmental disabilities and fewer social skills—and it gets worse with age. In childhood, efforts are made, but by the time kids hit age ten or so, when cliques and social circles form outside of parental control, ostracism and isolation are nearly complete.

In Canada, we talk a good game about integration, about breaking down barriers to allow the inclusion of people with physical and developmental disabilities in every aspect of daily life. But reality is more stark and harsh. Real integration requires a lot more than building ramps, adopting human rights legislation and funding programs. Grudging accommodation, with a dash of tokenism, is not enough. If we want people to be healthy—physically, mentally, emotionally—and to reach their full potential, they need to be full citizens. Kids with disabilities can't be segregated and shut out of mainstream society.

They need to be like every kid, in school, in swim class, on the bus, in the playground and hanging out at the mall with friends.

That is the underlying theme of Snowdon's report, *Strengthening Communities for Canadian Children with Disabilities*, which she presented at the annual conference of the Sandbox Project in January 2012. (Sandbox, founded in 2009 by pediatric surgeon and MP Kellie Leitch, is designed to spur improvements in the health outcomes of Canadian children in areas such as injury prevention, obesity, mental health and the environment.) "Children and youth with disabilities and their families need and want to connect and engage with their communities in a meaningful, accessible and accommodating way that enables social interaction and development," Snowdon said.

To conduct the research, Snowdon and her team did in-depth interviews with 166 families in Regina, Fredericton and Toronto, along with some focus groups. All the families had children with physical and developmental disabilities ranging from Down syndrome to autism. Children with psychiatric disabilities such as bipolar disorder were not included, but one can imagine the issues would be similar. Above all, the report focused on the practical. What are the challenges caregivers face and what help is available to them? Interestingly, the most common complaint was not lack of services but poor communication. "Finding information on what is available is a big challenge," said Sally Jordan, a caregiver to her twenty-two-year-old nephew with severe developmental disabilities. In this, the communications age, she relies on word-of-mouth and tips from other parents to find out what services are available.

As far as anyone can tell, a plethora of programs is available for kids with disabilities. But a startling 78 percent of parents said their children don't participate regularly in community programs—for a variety of reasons. Many programs are inaccessible (that doesn't mean there are no ramps; it means they are at inconvenient times or in inconvenient places). Transportation is a major problem for children who, because of their disabilities, can't use public transit. And cost is a big factor, especially as parents of children with lifelong disabilities often stop paid work to become caregivers.

In her report, Snowdon makes three main recommendations:

- Create a single online reference tool that lists all community programs, services and professional care available to people with disabilities.
- Invest in programs where disabled kids are integrated, not segregated, so they can feel they are part of their community.
- Find ways to expand the social networks of children and teenagers to break the isolation.

Facebook and other social networking tools have drawbacks, but they've been a godsend for many disabled kids because they remove barriers—like being judged for the way you look. But being a "virtual" citizen is only a baby step in the right direction—it's not enough. Snowdon said she was surprised to learn from both parents and children that isolation was far more painful to live with than physical or development disabilities themselves. It's an issue, she said, that really tugs at the heartstrings.

But beyond the emotional response, there are practical consequences. Social interaction is key to quality of life: it's how we find love, how we find work and how we have fun. Having a disability does not obviate those needs; if anything, it magnifies them. Sometimes we need to stop and reflect on the value of friendship, of a sense of belonging, and the value of community itself to our individual and collective health. Relationships matter more than fancy programs. To quote Mother Teresa, "Loneliness is the most terrible poverty."

—⟋⎸⟍—

Disabled workers need respect, not pity

In March 2015, the federal government ended a long-standing contract for document shredding, throwing fifty people out of work. In this era of cuts, pink slips for a few dozen paper-pushers wouldn't normally merit much notice. But the move sparked outrage because all the workers have intellectual and development disabilities, and some had been doing the work for as long as thirty-five years. So, shortly after, in a bid to limit the political fallout, the government reversed itself and extended the contract for three more years.

Ending the contract was dumb. Extending it was worse. What these workers—who by all accounts do their jobs well—need is not pity, but respect. They need to be afforded the same rights as other Canadians, including the protection of the country's labour laws. Under the paper-shredding contract, Library and Archives Canada pays the Ottawa-Carleton Association for Persons with Developmental Disabilities $124,600 a year. With that money, the OCAPDD operates a sheltered workshop, where its clients get work experience and are paid an "honorarium." The stipend is roughly $2,000 a year, the equivalent of $1.15 an hour. The minimum wage in Ontario is now $11.40 an hour; the only exceptions are students under eighteen and liquor servers (who depend on tips). There is no exception for people with disabilities, nor should there be.

Sheltered workshops come under many guises and euphemisms, such as "life skills," "training programs" and "employment training." They may be well intentioned, but they are outdated and counter-productive, a concept that the federal government should be working to eliminate, not perpetuate. People with disabilities deserve "real jobs for real pay," says Laurie Larson, president of the Canadian Association for Community Living.

What the two million Canadians living with disabilities—physical, psychiatric or developmental—want is to live up to their potential, to be full citizens like other Canadians. Having a job is good for your health. It not only provides income but helps build independence and self-esteem, especially for those who have been marginalized. Yet people with disabilities—most of whom can and want to work—have a horrendous unemployment rate, close to 50 percent.

According to a 2012 report, *Rethinking DisAbility in the Private Sector*, there are about 795,000 Canadians with disabilities who are able to work but are unemployed. The primary reason is prejudicial assumptions about ability to work and the cost of accommodation.

In fact, the report notes, hiring people with disabilities is good for business because it results in higher productivity, less turnover (which leads to lower training costs) and better responses from customers, who appreciate a workforce that reflects their community.

The paper-shredding workers all receive provincial disability benefits, which amount to about $800 to $1,000 a month. One of the reasons they are paid so little is that if they earn more than $200 a month, those payments are clawed back. This is a striking example of governments working at cross-purposes, and the dated condition of our approach to social welfare. Ottawa shouldn't be justifying exploitation by saying workers are receiving provincial benefits.

Instead of sheltered workshops that isolate people from mainstream society, workers with disabilities should be provided with supports for employment that help them integrate. A good example of this approach is Avalon Employment Inc. in St. John's, a nongovernmental organization that a) assists in the job search for people with barriers to employment, and b) helps employers find good workers. Avalon will, for example, help a person with Down syndrome or autism find work at a coffee shop and provide a co-worker to assist in training and skills building, at no cost to the employer. The workers are paid a wage like everyone else and the assistance usually isn't required for long. Doesn't that approach—integration, not isolation—make more sense, economic and otherwise, than the outmoded approach of sheltered workshops?

The Harper government had a pretty good record when it came to supporting people with disabilities, notably the creation of the innovative Registered Disability Savings Plan. It also actively promoted workplace diversity and encouraged employers to hire workers with disabilities. But Ottawa must do more. The good news is that the Liberal government has pledged to adopt a Canadians with Disabilities Act, legislation similar to the Americans with Disabilities Act, a labour law that prohibits unjustified discrimination based on disability and has had a dramatic impact on employment. Contracting workers in a sheltered workshop to work for a pittance instead of paying a decent living wage flies in the face of those policies and would no doubt violate a Canadians with disabilities law. That's a start, but to show real leadership, the federal government should embrace the Employment First concept, which promotes systemic change to fully integrate people with disabilities into the workplace.

The ultimate goal in a democracy should be to give everyone a voice and purpose. To do so, we need to build inclusive communities, from schools through to workplaces. We don't need antediluvian policies that relegate people with disabilities to second-class citizenship.

The amazing resilience of Canada's thalidomiders

There is nothing quite like a dance floor overflowing with people with missing arms and legs, on crutches, in wheelchairs, tripping the light fantastic with their parents, their children, their friends, even their lobbyists and lawyers. Yet the surreal scene, which unfolded one Saturday night in June 2016 at a hotel in Gatineau, Quebec, came as no surprise because nothing quite compares with Canada's thalidomiders. The victims—nay, survivors—of one of the country's worst medical disasters have always shown unbelievable resilience and grace in their fifty-year fight for justice, and it was on full display as they celebrated.

Thalidomide, a drug developed by the Nazis as an antidote for nerve gas during the Second World War, was marketed after the war as a "miracle drug" for treatment for morning sickness and insomnia, despite never having been properly tested, particularly on pregnant women. It was available in Canada from 1959 to 1962 under the brand names Kevadon and Talimol. The drug caused horrific limb deformities, damage to vital organs and miscarriages; in Canada, it remained on the shelves even after these dangers became clear. Worldwide, more than six thousand children were left with limb deformities caused by thalidomide. No one counted the tens of thousands of miscarriages.

Yet in the United States, no cases appeared because a single official, Canadian Dr. Frances Kelley, recognized that the drug was inadequately tested and should not be approved.

When the full extent of the egregious failings of the manufacturer and regulator became clear, it led to a complete revamp of drug safety laws in Canada. But victims and their families never received anything but token amounts of compensation, never mind an apology. Thalidomiders were essentially relegated to society's scrap heap, burdened by stigma, physical woes and often crushing poverty. But a few years back, aging survivors, of which there were fewer than one hundred in Canada, decided to make one last push for recognition and reparations. Against all odds, they won that battle—in both the court of public opinion and in Parliament—and received a $180 million settlement.

In the initial year of the deal, members of the Thalidomide Victims Association of Canada received their first payments—a $125,000 lump sum each, to be followed by annual compensation of between $25,000 and $100,000, depending on the severity of injuries. The money has been liberating and transformative, especially when you consider that, before the payouts, the average income of surviving thalidomiders was $14,000 a year. Individuals have purchased everything from homes to home care with their money; one survivor splurged modestly on a new mattress to help relieve his lifelong back pain. But they also wanted to celebrate as a group, so they organized a gala.

Mercedes Benegbi, the irrepressible leader of TVAC, opened the event in her inimitable fashion, with a piercing *cri de joie*. When she was born in Montreal in 1962, stunted and with flipper-like arms, a priest performed last rites, assuming she would soon die. But Benegbi's parents nurtured her instead of abandoning her, as other babies were, and she became the public face of thalidomide in Canada and a tireless advocate for justice. It was Benegbi who, in 2013, approached US lawyer Stephen Raynes—whose father had sued and won settlements for some thalidomide victims in the 1970s—to help. He embraced the cause and enlisted Canadian allies, including lawyer Joe Fiorante and well-known political lobbyist Barry Campbell. Together, they fashioned one of the most effective lobbying efforts in Canadian history, and they did it all pro bono, with little public recognition. (From the outset, they agreed that only thalidomide survivors would speak publicly.)

At their gala, the survivors generously honoured all these back-room players for their roles, along with *Globe and Mail* reporter Ingrid Peritz, who wrote a series of forceful stories in 2014 that pushed the struggle into the public spotlight, which resulted in a unanimous parliamentary vote on compensation on December 1, 2014. What they really should have celebrated was their own courage—the decision, after years of being stared at, mocked and dismissed, to risk putting themselves out there and telling their stories in a bid to put a human face on a public-policy failing.

The most remarkable aspect of the gala was its celebratory tone; not the slightest hint of anger or bitterness could be detected despite the decades of neglect thalidomide sufferers endured. "Nothing can totally correct the wrong inflicted on thalidomide victims. But today we have a balm on our wounds," Benegbi said.

There was virtually no talk of money either. Rather, the survivors spoke emotionally of how their fellow citizens no longer look upon them in horror, but with compassion. The victims of thalidomide were liberated not so much by money as by the acknowledgement of their self-worth—the formal recognition that they were wronged and that Canadian society had a duty to right that wrong. "What we have, after all these years, is our dignity," Benegbi said. That and the new-found confidence to let their hair down and dance with abandon. And dance they did.

CHAPTER 10

Indigenous Health

First Nations health care is
a sickening disgrace

A mad scientist, hell-bent on destroying the health of a population, could probably not imagine a more diabolical plan than this one. Take disparate groups of nomads, plunk them on land nobody else wants. Pack them like sardines into shoddy houses that become mould infested. Don't bother too much with infrastructure—just dump sewage in the river where people draw their water. Strip away language and cultural heritage and ship the kids to faraway residential schools so family life disintegrates. Don't concern yourself with employment—it's easier to create dependency with government handouts that ensure people remain poor. Make health-care services hard to access. Ensure even care for something as elemental as giving birth is a plane ride away. Keep food scarce and expensive. Subsidize only alcohol. Create an environment so unpalatable that drug abuse, criminality and suicide seem like the most appealing options in a young person's life. If people complain and the situation becomes so dire outsiders start paying attention, throw a few bucks the residents' way to quiet them until the media leave town.

Of course, would-be Dr. Evils need not trouble themselves with plotting because this diabolical reality already exists for the 4 percent of the Canadian population of indigenous ancestry—and not just on the Attawapiskat reserve in northern Ontario. The health status of the more than 1.4 million First Nations, Métis and Inuit peoples living in more than six hundred neglected and largely isolated communities (not to mention the inner cities of larger urban centres) is a national disgrace.

In Canada, we frown on collecting race-based statistics, ostensibly because we believe in equality. But where race-based statistics do exist regarding First Nations people, they tell a sickening tale of inequality. In 2016, the Canadian Centre for Policy Alternatives published a report titled *Shameful Neglect: Indigenous Child Poverty in Canada* that provides a grim reminder that indigenous children live in far worse conditions, economic and otherwise, than non-indigenous children, with poverty rates averaging 60 percent on reserves.

But poverty is just one measure. Over the years, countless studies and reports have exposed the dire state of population health among indigenous peoples. It makes for a mind-numbing collection of statistics:

- *Life expectancy:* Canadians have one of the world's highest life expectancies but indigenous people can expect to live about fifteen years less for men and ten years less for women, on average.
- *Disability:* Not only do indigenous people die younger, they live far longer with disabilities, about twelve more years on average.
- *Infant mortality:* First Nations children die at three times and Inuit children at five times the rate of other Canadian kids, and are more likely to be born with severe birth defects and debilitating conditions such as fetal alcohol syndrome.
- *Injuries:* Members of First Nations suffer traumatic injuries at four times the rate of the general population. Per capita, natives suffer more motor vehicle crashes, drownings, deaths by fire, homicide, accidental poisonings and firearms-related injuries.
- *Suicide:* Their rate is six times higher than other Canadians.
- *Chronic disease:* First Nations have three times the rate of diabetes; they suffer more heart disease and at a younger age. While cancer is one of the few diseases where the rate is lower, that is likely because so many natives die young, before they have a chance to get cancer.

- *Infectious disease:* Tuberculosis rates are sixteen times higher in First Nations than in the rest of Canada; HIV-AIDS rates are growing fastest in the native population; medieval water-borne illnesses like dysentery and shigellosis are still commonplace in native communities.

And that's just the obvious stuff. We know that the key determinants of health—individually and collectively—are social and economic factors such as housing, income, education, environment and empowerment. There, the record in First Nations, Métis and Inuit communities (three discrete groups) is even more dismal.

The unemployment and poverty rates are three times those in the non-indigenous community. Only 4 percent of First Nations people have a university education, one-quarter the rate in mainstream society. More than one-third have, in government jargon, a "core housing need," meaning their homes do not meet the most basic standard of acceptability. Overcrowding, lack of running water and inadequate sewage are the norm in many indigenous communities. The environmental contaminants that stalk some communities are frightening: mercury, PCBs, toxaphene and pesticide levels are all higher in the bodies of indigenous peoples than in non-indigenous peoples.

It is, all told, a "perfect storm" of conditions to destroy the health—and the soul—of a population. Misery has bred ill health, and ill health more misery. Throughout our history, we have tried to deal with the indigenous "problem" in almost every conceivable way: mass slaughter, the deliberate spread of infectious disease, displacement, the apartheid-like reserve system, assimilation and, more recently, Third-World health outcomes brought on by benign neglect. Perhaps the time has come to try sound public-health policy.

First Nations babies are refugees in their own land

The cornerstone of maternal and child care in many indigenous communities in Canada is uprooting women and sending them to big-city hospitals. At around thirty-six weeks of gestation—sometimes sooner if complications arise, such as diabetes, anemia or obesity—mothers-to-be are flown (or otherwise transported) hundreds, sometimes thousands, of kilometres away from home.

Birthing is not a mechanical act. Birthing is a physical, emotional, even spiritual experience. If there is a moment in her life when a woman does not want to be alone, a time when she needs to be close to her partner, her family, her other children and her friends, it is at birth. Yet, all too often, pregnant indigenous women are utterly alone, in strange, sterile white surroundings, where no one speaks their language, where the food is alien and where their only company is the kicking little bundle in their belly.

The indigenous community has a disproportionately large number of young mothers. Alone in a medical boarding home, a rooming house or a cut-rate hotel, too many pass the time waiting for the birth by partying—drinking and taking drugs. (The troubling rates of fetal alcohol syndrome and other birth defects in First Nations children are graphic testament to these social ills.) What should be a joyful occasion can become a frightfully lonely, self-destructive experience, one in which the precious child becomes detritus. Further, where women stay, who (if anyone) can accompany them to a birth, where the birth itself will take place, and when mother and baby will be shipped back home again all depend on a dizzying array of conditions—the band council's budget, provincial health policies, federal non-insured health benefits and even the weather. And in some cases, births are induced or Caesareans are performed to get mothers in and out of hospital quicker, a practice so common it has a name in First Nations communities—geographic inducement.

Can any mother reading this fathom being treated that way? Can any woman in Canada in 2017 imagine having to hold a bake sale, or begging for money outside the co-op store to raise enough cash to fly out to a hospital to give birth because the band council has exhausted its transport budget? That practice, too, has a name: canvassing. Is it possible to imagine a more alienating, discomforting manner in which to bring a child into the world than what so many First Nations women must endure? Yet the sordid scenario is repeated thousands of times a year in Canada.

When we wonder about the sorry state of indigenous health, we need look no further than maternal care for an understanding. Healthy people create healthy communities, and healthy communities beget healthy people. When women are separated from the support of their families and friends, there is an increased risk of premature birth, and of maternal and newborn complications. All-too-common chronic conditions such as diabetes, and lifestyle issues such as smoking, drinking and poor nutrition, magnify that risk. Women who experience the stress of faraway birth with little support are more likely to suffer postpartum depression and less likely to breastfeed successfully. Not to mention that many First Nations mothers now worry about breastfeeding because of the high levels of mercury, PCBs and other toxins in their milk.

Pregnant indigenous women are caught in a terrible Catch-22: an investment needs to be made in locally delivered health care, including maternal care and birthing services such as midwives, but an increasing number are now high-risk moms and need to be med-evaced out because the potential complications pose too great a risk. First Nations mothers-to-be are also caught in the centre of a nasty federal–provincial spat: Ottawa is happy to pay for transport out of First Nations communities because the cost of health-care delivery then has to be assumed by the provinces. As a result, patients—and the high number of birthing mothers in particular—are not made to feel particularly welcome. In a bid to avoid all this nastiness, some women do not show up at the nursing station until their cervix is dilated to ten centimetres, making transport out too risky. They call this the ten-centimetre strategy. But this desperate bid to birth at home can be risky, too.

The petty political bickering needs to stop. The vicious circle of poor care resulting in the need for even more care must be broken. If there is going to be any hope of improving the health—physical, economic, spiritual—of Canada's 1.4 million indigenous people, we have to start with the babies. For the healing to begin, babies—with few exceptions—must be born close to home, into loving families and nurturing communities. We cannot afford or tolerate another generation of First Nations, Inuit and Métis children entering the world as refugees in their own land.

---||---

Tribunal decision is a legal and moral victory for First Nations children

On January 26, 2016, the Canadian Human Rights Tribunal (CHRT) ruled that First Nations children were victims of wilful and reckless discrimination by the federal government. Specifically, it said funding formulas used by Aboriginal Affairs and Northern Development Canada—which resulted in social-service programs on reserves receiving funding that was between 22 and 34 percent less than equivalent programs off-reserve—were a violation of human rights. This is an important legal and moral victory, especially for First Nations children. As tribunal members Sophie Marchildon and Edward Lustig write in the opening words of their ruling, "This decision concerns children. More precisely, it is about how the past and current child welfare practices in First Nations communities on reserves, across Canada, have impacted and continue to impact First Nations children, their families and their communities."

What the tribunal exposed is that, despite all the soothing words and flowery promises that have followed inquiries like the Truth and Reconciliation Commission and the Royal Commission on Aboriginal Peoples, institutional racism is still the daily reality at the highest levels of government. If you think that is overstating the case, consider that it took nine long years to get a ruling on what is clearly a glaring injustice. What possible justification could there be for saying that indigenous kids and their parents deserve one-third less for social services, particularly given that a) welfare payments are already pitifully low, b) social supports are more often a crying need on-reserve than off, and c) life on the rez is costly.

The federal government, throughout the interminable process, never once argued that its practices were good for children. Rather, it bogged down the process in beside-the-point bureaucratic arguments about jurisdiction and the like. To make matters worse, the former Conservative government even resorted to McCarthyesque tactics to discredit the principal complainant in the case, Dr. Cindy Blackstock of the First Nations Child & Family Caring Society. She was spied on, shut out of meetings and denied jobs for which she was qualified, all in retaliation for making a human rights complaint. This whole sorry tale was revealed in a previous CHRT ruling, in which Blackstock was awarded $20,000. (She donated the money to children's charities.) As NDP MP Charlie Angus said, "Cindy Blackstock is one of the great civil rights heroines of our nation." The tribunal ruling is a vindication for her.

But Blackstock will be the first to say that no moral victory and no amount of money can undo the damage done by entrenched, deleterious social-welfare policies. Because of "funding formulas," many children were denied proper care and many parents were denied a livable income. Many parents also lost custody of their children at least in part because of the inadequacy and underfunding of services. Some children, like Jordan River Anderson, even died while Ottawa and provinces bickered over who should pay for care and how much. This gave rise to a policy known as Jordan's Principle that holds that the "government of first contact" pay for services and then seek reimbursement later. In other words, put the welfare of children first, and jurisdiction disputes a distant second.

These are not trivial matters for 163,000 First Nations children and their parents and guardians who live on-reserve and under federal jurisdiction. We can no longer make the mistake of dismissing this as bureaucratic nickel-and-diming because it's much more. It's a continuation of racist (and, in some cases, genocidal) policies like the Indian Act, residential schools and the Sixties Scoop (the 1960s through 1980s practice of "scooping" First Nations children from their families and placing them in foster homes or for adoption). More indigenous children are in foster care and other forms of state care today than were ever in residential schools and; in many cases, the cultural dislocation and the abuse, psychological and sexual, are just as bad. Have we learned nothing from our shameful history?

The Canadian Human Rights Tribunal ruling suggests strongly that we have not learned enough. So how do we begin to fix it? The CHRT, in its ruling, did not rule on compensation. The Caring Society has asked that every First Nations child be awarded the maximum $20,000 each. More importantly, the tribunal has the power to order government to end its discriminatory practices, and that could have profound repercussions. As Marchildon and Lustig write in their ruling, "More than just funding, there is a need to refocus the policy of the program to respect human rights principles and sound social work practice. In the best interest of the child, all First Nations children and families living on-reserve should have an opportunity '… equal with other individuals to make for themselves the lives that they are able and wish to have and to have their needs accommodated, consistent with their duties and obligations as members of society.'"

If Canada and its government truly believe in human rights for all, indigenous people cannot be second-class citizens, in policy or in practice.

Indigenous children bear
the brunt of poverty

In 2016, Canada was home to 6.9 million children, 1.2 million of whom live in poverty. That's 18 percent. That number is bad enough in itself, but it becomes even more disturbing when you consider that, within the subset of 478,000 indigenous children in the country, 182,000 live in poverty. That's 38 percent. Of course, these numbers from a 2016 report by the Canadian Centre for Policy Alternatives (titled *Shameful Neglect: Indigenous Child Poverty in Canada*) tell us something we already knew: indigenous children live in far worse conditions, economic and otherwise, than non-indigenous children.

But no matter how inured we become to that grim reality, the numbers are worth pondering because they are a sharp reminder that, even in a country such as Canada that takes pride in its multiculturalism and diversity, a person's health status is profoundly influenced by his or her racial/ethnic identity and geography. Slicing the CCPA data in various ways to examine it from different angles reveals the following range of poverty rates among Canadian children:

· for First Nations living on-reserve, the rate is 60 percent;
· First Nations living off-reserve, 41 percent;
· First Nations with "status," 51 percent;
· non-status First Nations, 29 percent;
· Inuit, 25 percent;
· Métis, 23 percent;
· immigrants, 32 percent;
· visible minorities, 22 percent; and
· non-immigrant, non-racialized (read: Caucasian), 13 percent.

The focus of the report, rightly, is on the children among the more than 1.4 million people in Canada who identify as indigenous, about

4 percent of the population. Half of that total are "registered Indians," 30 percent are Métis, 15 percent are non-status Indians and 4 percent are Inuit. More than half of indigenous people live in urban centres. These figures are a lot to digest, but they should, nonetheless, be the object of much reflection for our politicians and policy-makers. They are, among other things, an eloquent illustration of the fact that Canadian society is stratified by class, by race and by income, a direct challenge to our comfy belief that we are an egalitarian, socially progressive and colour-blind country. What we look like and where we came from have an inarguable impact on our opportunities, our income and our health.

So does where we live. Again, the CCPA report reminds us not only that child poverty is widespread, but there is a geography of poverty. The poorest of the poor are found predominantly in the country's 617 First Nations communities, most of them reserves established by the Indian Act of 1876. Many of these communities are small and isolated—out of sight and out of mind. They also, for the most part, have abysmal health and social services, a situation made worse by the fact that the federal government openly discriminates by funding on-reserve services at levels 22 percent to 34 percent lower than those off-reserve. (While the Canadian Human Rights Tribunal recently ordered the federal government to fix this, it has yet to do so.)

As well, important disparities between the provinces exist: in Manitoba, 76 percent of on-reserve First Nations children live in poverty; First Nations kids living off-reserve fare better—if you can actually consider Winnipeg's 42 percent rate of child poverty laudable. One of the few bright spots—again, all things being relative—is the Eeyou Istchee (James Bay Cree), where the child poverty rate is relatively low at 23 percent. It is not a coincidence that the communities there are highly autonomous and have modern treaties that allow them to benefit from the exploitation of natural resources on their territory, including hydro dams, forestry and mining. By contrast, across the bay in Ontario's Attawapiskat—which was in the news because of its suicide crisis—the child poverty rate is 48 percent, and there is no revenue sharing with the nearby diamond mine or forestry companies.

The CCPA report offers some well-worn recommendations to address the problem of rampant indigenous child poverty: better tracking of the data, improving income supports, bolstering employment opportunities and implementing long-term solutions. That last recommendation is the key to ending the shameful neglect. The long road out of poverty and despair begins with reconciliation and self-government and, in the words of the Truth and Reconciliation Commission, "unlocking the potential of First Nations to improve the lives of their own citizens, including their children."

CHAPTER II

Cancer

Cancer: The name that can hurt you

Hippocrates, the father of Western medicine, gave cancer its name. He used the words *carcinos* and *carcinoma* to describe tumours—Greek words for "crab." At the time, around 400 BC, cancer was discovered in the end stage, when tumours were a hard mass, like a crab's shell. The sharp pain of end-stage cancer that patients described also reminded Hippocrates of the pinch of a crab's claw. He thought cancer was caused by black bile (one of the four bodily fluids believed responsible for all illness), a theory that was accepted into the seventeenth century, when scientists began to understand the circulatory and lymphatic systems. It wasn't until the late nineteenth century that Rudolph Virchow recognized that cancerous cells divide uncontrollably and invade other tissues by spreading through the blood and lymphatic system.

We know now that cancer is not one disease but many diseases that have their origins in a complex mix of genetics, lifestyle factors and triggers (ranging from smoking to poverty). Still, the number-one risk factor remains aging, which is why cancer kills more people today than it ever has, with public-health measures such as sanitation having dramatically reduced infectious-disease deaths. There are hundreds of different types of cancer, most of which are named for the organ or type of cell in which they start. We also know that not all tumours are cancerous—they can be malignant (spreading to other parts of the body) or benign (they do not spread). Some cancers, like leukemia, do not even form tumours at all. Further, thanks to technological advances, we can now detect tumours at a microscopic level and abnormalities right down to a cellular level—and we can do so in living people. (For the longest time, cancer was studied only in corpses, reinforcing the notion of deadliness.) The paradox is that we can now detect a lot of cancer that is, well, not even cancer yet and likely never will be.

In the fall of 2016, the Canadian Cancer Society estimated that 78,800 Canadians would die of cancer that year, while approximately 202,400 new cases of cancer would be diagnosed in Canada. For every one of those people, the cancer diagnosis will pack a punch. When you get a diagnosis of cancer, the assumption is that you're going to suffer and you're going to die prematurely. But for many, many "cancers," that simply isn't true anymore. So, should we be telling folks with abnormalities or weird-looking cells that they have cancer? This is a question that health professionals, activists and patients themselves are increasingly struggling with.

Essentially, we need a new cancer lexicon—one in which the language reflects the knowledge of the twenty-first century, not the fears of 400 BC. The Canadian Cancer Society, in its annual tally of cancer diagnoses, excludes all non-melanoma skin cancers because they are localized abnormalities. Given evolving scientific knowledge, it may well be time to start making that distinction for some forms of breast, prostate and thyroid "cancers."

Research published in the medical journal *JAMA Oncology* in August 2015 noted that one-quarter of the 25,700 breast cancer cases in Canada were classified as ductal carcinoma in situ (DCIS), also known as Stage 0 breast cancer. Increasingly, it is being asked, is DCIS actually cancer at all? Sure, it's not always benign; it can spread from the milk ducts to elsewhere, but no good evidence exists to show that treating it before it spreads is beneficial. The mortality rate is the same whether a woman undergoes treatment—lumpectomy or mastectomy, with or without radiation—or not. A panel of experts from the US National Institutes of Health concluded that DCIS is not a carcinoma, so it should be renamed high-grade dysplasia. That distinction already exists in the cervical cancer field, where cervical carcinoma in situ (in the body) was renamed cervical intraepithelial neoplasia. Women understand too that an abnormal Pap test does not automatically mean they have cancer; they make the distinction between dysplasia and cancer.

The fastest-growing cancer in Canada is thyroid cancer. But again, that is misleading. As with DCIS, we now have technology that can detect nodules on the thyroid. But the great majority are benign—they will have no negative health consequences, unless you start cutting them out. Is that really cancer?

Language matters because it influences behaviour. When you use the dreaded C-word, the reaction of patients is to want to rid their body of a deadly passenger. They want to cut it out—whether it's in a breast, a prostate or a thyroid. But cutting and burning and poisoning—surgery, radiation and chemotherapy if you prefer the more technical terms—are not always the best response to weird-looking cells.

Watchful waiting is becoming an increasingly common practice, particularly with prostate cancer, where the screening test (PSA or prostate-specific antigen) is notoriously poor and tumour growth often very slow. The severity of prostate cancer is determined using something called Gleason scoring. The physician who created this system, Donald Gleason, has suggested that the most common tumours (Gleason 3 + 3) actually be renamed adenosis, a term used to describe benign swelling. Prostate cancer is sometimes described as a cancer you die with, not a cancer you die from. We are learning that this is true of many other "cancers." Increasingly, we have the ability to make those distinctions, and we should do so.

We do ourselves a disservice when conditions as wildly different as a grade 4 glioblastoma multiforme (a brain tumour that is virtually 100 percent fatal) and prostatic intraepithelial neoplasia (a condition more likely to make you pee often than kill you) are both described as cancer. Hippocrates is best known not for his naming of cancer but his admonition to physicians to, above all, do no harm. Right now, our crude, imprecise use of the term *cancer* is doing harm. The words we use need to reflect our knowledge, and influence practice.

Does breast cancer
screening save lives?

"Breast cancer screening saved my life" is one of the most power-ful narratives in modern medicine, if not in Western culture more generally. For the past generation, as breast cancer survivors and their loved ones built a powerful social movement, a couple of key messages have been hammered home: 1) breast cancer is a major killer of women, and 2) spotting cancer early with screening is your best defence. But in the enthusiastic push to inform and empower—most of it well-meaning, but some of it commercially driven—those messages have become perverted. It is fine to embrace pink ribbons, walks for the cure and the like, but not at the expense of science and context. So, first and foremost, women need a bit of a reality check.

Yes, breast cancer is a major killer. About 25,000 women (and 220 men) were diagnosed with breast cancer in 2015. Approximately 5,000 Canadian women (and 60 men) died of breast cancer. The deaths oc-curred overwhelmingly in women in their seventies and eighties. That is not to suggest they are unimportant, but we will all die of something, mostly diseases of aging like cancer and cardiovascular disease.

Many scary statistics are trotted out, but the bottom line is this: the average woman has a 3 percent lifetime risk of dying of breast cancer. Breasts are not ticking time bombs and young women, with few exceptions, are not dying of breast cancer. Still, if we can prevent women (and men) from developing breast cancer, if we can minimize their suffering by delaying the onset of symptoms, if we can extend survival in cancer sufferers with better treatments, we should. But how do we do so?

In recent years, the philosophy we embraced was to spot a cancer-ous tumour early, eliminate it (with surgery, radiation or chemother-apy), and cancer would be beaten and mortality reduced. We invested heavily in screening: mass mammography screening programs were developed and promoted. In Canada, more than four million women get mammograms annually, at a cost of about $500 million. Women have also been urged to do routine breast self-examination (BSE) at the same time every month; and physicians and nurses have been trained in clinical breast examination.

But over time, research has shown that the mantra "early detection saves lives" is flawed and that screening is not the lifesaver it is made out to be. In fact, one of the largest studies ever conducted, where ninety thousand women were followed over twenty-five years—with half randomly assigned to be screened or not—found there was no impact on mortality at all, and a modest impact on survival. (The distinction here is important: woman survive longer because they are diagnosed earlier, but they don't live longer. Scientists call this phenomenon lead-time bias.) Studies have shown similarly disappointing results for BSE and clinical breast exams.

The current breast cancer screening guidelines, drafted by the Canadian Task Force on Preventive Health Care, reflect the science, and as a result they are immensely unpopular. Given the grumbling since their publication in 2011, it's worth repeating what the guidelines actually say, not what critics—and, to a lesser extent, supporters—say they say:

1) The task force said women aged fifty to seventy-four should have screening mammograms every two to three years. (In many provinces, screening is still offered annually beginning at age forty.) The task force did not reject screening mammography. Rather, it said screening works best in postmenopausal women, with the caveats that more is not better and earlier is not better.

2) Routine clinical breast examinations and breast self-examination are no longer recommended because they do more harm than good. The task force did not say women should not be aware of changes in their breasts; on the contrary, it noted that more than half of cancers are detected in this manner. What it said is that doing systematic checks—examining your

breasts each month at the same point in your menstrual period, as used to be counselled—confers no real benefit.

These recommendations, of course, do not apply to high-risk women—for example, those with a personal or family history of breast cancer or who have tested positive for the breast cancer genes BRCA1 or BRCA2.

One important aspect of screening that is too often glossed over is that it can do harm. Research shows that, over a ten-year period, one in every two women who get routine mammograms will receive a false positive. Aside from the psychological impact of a cancer scare, one in eleven women diagnosed with breast cancer will get treatment that is unnecessary—undergoing biopsies, radiation and surgery.

Paradoxically, it tends to be healthy young women—those who will benefit least and suffer the greatest harms—who tend to be most assiduous. The reality is that women are more likely to be overdiagnosed and overtreated than actually helped by the test. As Dr. Susan Love, the breast cancer pioneer (and supporter of screening over age fifty), is fond of reminding us: "All too often, when it comes to breast cancer, we seem to get caught up in wishful thinking and forget about science."

—/\—

Found: A c-word for cancer

There is a Run for the Cure, a Ride to Conquer Cancer and a Weekend to End Women's Cancers (which was changed in 2016 to OneWalk to Conquer Cancer), among others; these fundraising events have catchy names that tell of lofty goals. But how much cancer can we really cure and conquer, and can we realistically hope to eradicate breast cancer, or any other cancer for that matter?

Canadians are surviving cancer more often and longer than ever before. There are a couple of common ways of measuring this. The five-year relative survival rate for all cancers combined is 59 percent; this means that those diagnosed with cancer are 59 percent as likely to live for another five years as are comparable members of the general population who are cancer free. The more common way of measuring is calculating what percentage of people are alive five years after diagnosis. Those five-year survival rates vary widely depending on type of cancer, from a dismal 6 percent for pancreatic cancer to a remarkable 95 percent for thyroid, prostate and testicular cancers. For the most common cancers, the rates vary, too: lung, 17 percent; colorectal, 64 percent; breast, 87 percent; and prostate, 95 percent.

But these numbers do not distinguish between those who will die of cancer and those who will not. With advances in early detection, treatment and care, patients don't merely survive cancer any more—they can be cured. Yet many clinicians and researchers avoid the c-word, *cure*, because it implies some sort of miracle that came about through divine intervention. Speaking of cures can also give some patients unrealistic expectations. But being cured simply means that, after treatment, a patient's life expectancy is identical to that of a comparable member of the general population. Put another way, their relative survival rate is 100 percent for five years and beyond. This means they will die of something other than their primary cancer.

Research published in the September 2015 edition of the *European Journal of Cancer* offers detailed numbers on how many people are cured of cancer. Not surprisingly, the numbers vary widely by type of cancer and by country. Across the thirty-one European countries participating in the Eurocare-5 study, 5 to 14 percent of lung cancer patients were cured; between 11 and 35 percent were cured of stomach cancer; 40 to 66 percent were cured of colorectal cancer; and 69 to 87 percent were cured of breast cancer. In the latter two, high cure rates were attributed principally to screening, the implication being that when a cancer is diagnosed early, it is more treatable and hence more curable. (The problem with early detection is that it creates lead-time bias—meaning people survive longer after diagnosis, but with no improvement in life expectancy. But the European numbers that focus on cure rather than five-year survival suggest genuine progress in controlling cancer.)

The research also shows, not too surprisingly, that survival and cure rates in the elderly (defined as those over seventy) with cancer were worse than among the middle-aged (fifty-five to sixty-nine) and that women of all ages respond better to cancer treatment than men do, which suggests that sex hormones play a role. Finally, the Eurocare-5 study—with data on more than twenty million cancer patients collected since 1978, it is one of the most extensive data collections in the world—demonstrates that survival and cure rates have risen steadily for two decades, offering a lot of hope to those diagnosed with cancer.

In 2016, an estimated 202,400 Canadians were diagnosed with cancer, and about 78,800 died of cancer. About 42 percent of women and 45 percent of men will develop cancer during their lifetimes, and about one in four Canadians can expect to die of it. That cancer numbers continue to rise is, in some ways, a success story. After all, cancer is largely a disease (or, more precisely, a vast array of diseases) of aging. Many people now live long enough to get cancer. The new data remind us that, particularly at a younger age, we can cure many forms of cancer rather effectively. In Canada, more than 60 percent of people diagnosed with cancer can expect to survive more than five years after treatment, ranging from 17 percent for lung cancer to 95 percent for prostate cancer.

But improving survival (and cure) rates should not distract us from the fact that we can also prevent a lot of cancer, and prevention is a lot more effective (not to mention more pleasant) than treatment. A 2009 poll commissioned by the Canadian Partnership Against Cancer showed that close to half of Canadians (43 percent) believe a person's chance of developing cancer is based largely on the luck of the draw. In fact, cancer comes about as a combination of genetics, lifestyle and socio-economic circumstance. Just as a significant percentage of cancer can be cured if caught early, between one-quarter and one-third of all cancers worldwide can be prevented through lifestyle choices such as a healthy diet, regular physical activity and a healthy body weight, according to another international study.

So while Canadians walk, run and bike for a cure, they also need to remember they can walk, run and bike to prevent cancer in the first place. Prevention, treatment and cure should not be distinct entities, but parts of the same continuum of care, one that requires infrastructure, investment, sound public policies and personal awareness and commitment.

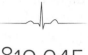

810,045

The annual publication *Cancer Statistics* is, as the name would suggest, largely a dry compilation of data. But behind every number is a story, few more compelling and complex than a number tucked away quietly on page seventy-four of the 2016 report. 810,045. That is the number of people who had been diagnosed with cancer in the previous ten years and were still alive on January 1, 2016.

It is astonishing to think that the number of cancer survivors in Canada today is equivalent to the population of a large city. Put another way, one in every forty-one Canadians have survived more than ten years after cancer diagnosis. Among this army of cancer survivors are 176,360 women who have battled breast cancer, 158,430 men who overcame prostate cancer, 105,195 people who survived colorectal cancer and even 39,350 women and men successfully treated for lung cancer.

There is no geographic breakdown of survivorship, but there should be. One of the dirty little secrets in Canada's health-care system is that the quality of treatment and care can vary markedly across different locations. In the cancer field, there is an unofficial postal-code lottery, in which patients in less populous, poorer areas of the country, such as the Atlantic region and the Far North, get short shrift. The Canadian Strategy for Cancer Control was created, in part, to address this disparity. The ambitious strategy aims to reduce the burden of cancer by preventing disease, detecting it early and ensuring that those stricken by it receive the best possible care, regardless of where they live.

The survivorship numbers remind us of the importance of this strategy. The numbers are growing annually because of earlier diagnosis and better treatment and because people are living longer. It's not all bad news, though there are still tens of thousands of cancer deaths annually. However, we should not fall into the trap of thinking that because the proliferation of cancerous cells has been stopped, a person can forget they had cancer. Nor can the health system behave as if the initial medical treatment of cancer is all that needs to be done. On the contrary, it is often just the beginning of a person's health-care journey. It is true that many—most, even, according to the stats—individuals who survive cancer will live productive and rewarding lives for many years after their diagnosis. Survivors make symbolic gestures such as dragon-boat racing and running for the cure, but they also work, volunteer and raise their families. But the cancer experience is never easy. The words "you have cancer" strike like a mace. Then treatment and survival present physical, emotional and spiritual challenges that can last years, even decades. Generally speaking, cancer treatments are not as disfiguring or debilitating as they used to be, but they are still no walk in the park. Treatment—which can consist of surgery, radiation, chemotherapy or some combination thereof—can last a year and sometimes much more.

In April 2009, *The Globe and Mail* featured the story of Shawn Sajkowski, who was diagnosed with non-Hodgkin's lymphoma at age twenty-five. His treatment lasted six years and included three relapses, nineteen rounds of chemotherapy and an arduous stem-cell transplant. Sajkowski also missed twenty months of work, had to move back home with his parents, and his long-term relationship collapsed under the strain. His story reminds us that cancer's tentacles reach far beyond the body.

The financial impact can also be staggering, especially for a person with cancer who does not have a job with a good short-term disability plan and extensive drug benefits. It can be even worse for parents of children with cancer, who often leave their jobs to be full-time care-givers and see debt pile up that adds to their stress. One of the biggest financial hardships is created by the lack of universal drug coverage under our current medicare scheme. Cancer drugs are covered when a patient is treated in hospital, but in many cases they have to be paid for privately (by private insurance or out-of-pocket) afterward. Drug coverage is particularly poor in the Atlantic provinces, putting cancer patients there at a distinct disadvantage.

The health system we have now, with its silos and its illogical disconnect with the social welfare system, is not equipped to deal with cancer survivors after a diagnosis. When oncology treatment stops, cancer survivors still have financial needs, may have mental-health challenges (depression is common), may require rehabilitation (especially if they have lost a limb or eyesight) and need regular medical monitoring. For some, cancer poses lifelong problems, while for others it can be episodic. Treatments can leave survivors infertile or cause secondary illnesses such as heart disease. Cancer survivors also have a high likelihood of developing a second cancer, often more aggressive than the first, a reality that can hang over their heads like the sword of Damocles.

Yet it is hard to find a family doctor in many parts of Canada. And general practitioners are not necessarily well versed in the needs of long-time cancer survivors. Survivors themselves have responded by creating all manner of support groups. But this does not replace the need for a human resources strategy. Simply put, Canada's health system is not prepared to deal with the large and ever-growing number of people living with cancer and other chronic illnesses.

The number 810,045 should give us pause. But counting cancer survivors is not enough. They need to be monitored and cared for properly. And with 42 percent of Canadian women and 45 percent of men expected to develop cancer during their lifetimes, it is a challenge all of us should demand be met.

The big cancer risk is the sun, not the cellphone

There has been much talk of late about the potential cancer risks posed by the radiation emitted from cellphones. Yet there is this big electromagnetic radiation transmitter in the sky whose risks we tend to ignore. It is called the sun.

The theoretical cancer risks posed by excessive cellphone use are minimal, despite the findings of a 2011 analysis from the International Agency for Research on Cancer (IARC). Jack Siemiatycki, who holds the Guzzo chair in environment and cancer research at the University of Montreal and is a member of the IARC expert panel, summarized the findings this way: "The meeting didn't determine that cellphones cause cancer. It didn't determine that they probably cause cancer. It determined they possibly cause cancer." There is no such vagueness in articulating the risks of excessive exposure to the sun; that it can cause cancer is undeniable and well demonstrated. Yet we fear cellphones more than we fear sunburn. This incongruity says a lot about our skewed perceptions of risk in modern society. And fearing the microwatts of cellphones more than the watts of the sun speaks to our lack of science literacy.

Microwaves, such as those emitted by cellphones, are non-ionizing radiation. They essentially produce heat. They can fry your brain if you crank them up to the level of a microwave oven, one-thousand-plus watts, but not at a few millionths of a watt, which a phone produces. Very little evidence exists that the radiation of cellphones can cause cellular damage. The risk is about the same as getting cancer from eating pickles. Sunshine consists largely of non-ionizing radiation as well. The sun kills immediately only when exposure is extreme, such as heatstroke. But the sun's rays also carry ionizing radiation, the kind that causes cellular damage that is at the root of cancer.

It goes without saying that the sun, unlike cellphones, is essential to life on Earth. Without the sun, we would be hard-pressed to produce food, and life would be dark and dreary. Direct exposure to the sun, and ultraviolet radiation in particular, is necessary to good health too; ultraviolet light stimulates the production of vitamin D, an essential nutrient. Lack of vitamin D is associated with some cancers and is likely a factor in autoimmune diseases such as multiple sclerosis. But all good things in moderation. For Caucasians, up to fifteen minutes of exposure to the sun, two to three times a week, is sufficient for adequate vitamin D synthesis, while darker-skinned individuals need slightly longer exposure. (In winter months, the sun's rays are too weak to produce vitamin D, so supplements are recommended.)

Skin cancer is by far the most common cancer. According to the Canadian Cancer Society, in 2014, an estimated 76,100 Canadians were diagnosed with non-melanoma skin cancers. In 2016, another 6,800 were diagnosed with more serious melanoma skin cancer. In 2016, melanoma killed an estimated 1,200 people in Canada; the non-melanoma (basal cell and squamous cell) cancers killed roughly 440 people. (The Cancer Society has stopped reporting detailed statistics on non-melanoma skin cancers because the data are imprecise: many cases are treated by family physicians and not reported to cancer registries.)

In the past thirty-five years, the incidence of skin cancer has risen threefold, the result of a combination of better surveillance, earlier detection and changes in diagnostic criteria, as well as changes in sun exposure behaviour and increases in ultraviolet exposure due to thinning of the ozone layer. In other words, while the sun is getting more dangerous, we're better at detecting skin cancer, and we're also seeing the consequences of our past follies, such as long days of sun-tanning on the beach and tanning beds. Skin cancer is also pricey, with treatment costs exceeding $500 million a year.

We've learned a lot in recent years about the nitty-gritty of risk. For example, a history of sunburn is a key measure of risk: a person who has suffered three sunburns in a decade has a threefold risk of developing melanoma (the most severe form of skin cancer) compared to someone with fewer burns. Levels of exposure in childhood and adolescence are good predictors of the risk of basal cell cancer. Squamous cell cancers—which tend to occur on exposed areas such as the face, neck and arms—follow a geographical pattern: they are most common in the sunniest parts of the world.

But we know how to protect ourselves from the cancer-causing rays of the sun. It is recommended by the Canadian Cancer Society, dermatologists and others that we limit our exposure to the sun, particularly during peak UV hours, use sunscreen and wear protective items such as hats, sunglasses and long sleeves. In recent years, important new sunscreen information has been published in both the United States and Britain. The US Food and Drug Administration, for example, unveiled new labelling rules in 2011 decreeing that for a sunscreen to state it can help prevent cancer, it must have a sun protection factor of at least 15 and protect against both UVA and UVB rays. The FDA had also said sunscreens cannot assert they are waterproof, just water-resistant, and claims of an SPF over 50 are not permitted.

The SPF is a measure of how much longer skin covered with a product takes to redden (or develop erythema, to use the scientific term) in response to UV radiation compared with unprotected skin. An SPF 15 sunscreen limits exposure to about 7 percent of UVB radiation, and an SPF 30 to about 3 percent. However, as the *British Drug and Therapeutics Bulletin* noted, those figures are based on the assumption that sunscreen is applied at a thickness of two milligrams for each square centimetre—a level at which it would run off the skin and be unsightly. In real life people apply much less, so you should assume that your SPF 30 sunscreen is offering no better than SPF 15 protection.

The point is this: we are exposed to various types of radiation all the time, from natural and man-made sources. We can protect ourselves from these exposures—and even benefit from some—but the key is to have a little basic scientific knowledge and apply it appropriately and practically in our daily lives.

———⊣⊢———

Research shows treatments are still driven by the assumption cancer has to be hit early and hard

In 2015, new Canadian research exposed the troubling reality that, for decades, we had probably been grossly overtreating early-stage breast cancer. In fact, ductal carcinoma in situ (DCIS)—a cluster of abnormal cells in the milk ducts—is probably not even cancer at all, though that's semantics. So what are women, and people worried about cancer more generally, supposed to take from this? Most importantly, this is progress. Painful, shocking, frustrating and confusing, perhaps, but progress nonetheless.

Despite the fact that cancer is one of the top killers in Western society—there were about 78,800 cancer deaths in Canada alone in 2016, including 4,900 breast cancer deaths—we still have a lot to learn about the biology, the genetics, the risk factors and skilful detection and treatment (and non-treatment) of the multitude of diseases we lump under the catch-all term *cancer*. Breast cancer is fairly common: an estimated 25,700 cases were diagnosed in Canada in 2016. About one-quarter of those cases will be classified as DCIS, or Stage 0 breast cancer. (There are five stages of cancer, from 0 to 4, based on the distance of spread from the point of origin, which is often a reflection of severity.) DCIS is an accumulation of abnormal-looking cells in the milk ducts of the breast. This condition was unknown before mammography screening because no lump can be felt, but the "weird cells" show up on X-rays. The 2015 study, led by Dr. Steven Narod of the Women's College Research Institute in Toronto, analyzed twenty years of data on 100,000 women diagnosed with DCIS. It found that 3.3 percent of DCIS patients died of breast cancer, regardless of their treatment—lumpectomy or mastectomy, with or without radiation. That is the same as the breast cancer mortality rate in the general population. This does not necessarily mean treatment was useless. But it does tell us that more aggressive treatment was not helpful and, in many cases, probably harmful.

Cancer is a word used to describe a malignant growth or tumour resulting from the abnormal division of cells. The notion that cells grow, spread out of control and become deadly has long been gospel, and this has led us to believe that the sooner we detect and treat cancerous cells the better. But in recent years, those fundamental beliefs have been challenged. In reality, abnormal cells appear all the time in the body. Some multiply quickly and do harm, even deadly harm; some spread ever so slowly, meaning you die with cancer, not of cancer; and some cancers can even regress or disappear, with or without treatment. In other words, not all cancers metastasize and kill. This has led to some new approaches to care, such as watchful waiting (also known as active surveillance) for men with prostate cancer. That means doing nothing—no surgery, no radiation, no chemotherapy—unless the cancer spreads.

Could watchful waiting be the proper approach to DCIS? Perhaps, though we have to be clear that, while the 2015 study suggests this, it does not demonstrate it. As counterintuitive as it may seem, doing little or nothing, even when a "cancer" is detected, is a legitimate clinical choice, and it is not valued nearly enough. As Dr. Otis Brawley, chief medical officer of the American Cancer Society, said, "Too often in medicine, we find something, we call it an illness and we overtreat it."

Before mammography, DCIS was virtually unknown, a condition seen only in autopsies. Advances in imaging technology have helped us see more—including lesions in milk ducts—but seeing does not necessarily mean understanding. An assumption was made that the clumps of abnormal cells dubbed DCIS were life-threatening and had to be treated aggressively. That assumption was wrong.

This should lead us to adjust treatment options, and also to some profound reflections, namely whether our population-wide screening programs are doing more harm than good. Too many of our policies—from screening to (over)treatment—are driven by fear, by the assumption that cancer is a savage killer that has to be hit early and hard. In the past century, we have become a lot better at detecting cancer and preventing recurrences. But mortality rates remain stubbornly steady. A key number in the 2015 study bears repeating: despite all our worries that breast cancer is a deadly scourge, only about one in twenty-nine will actually die of the condition. That's still too many. What we need more than anything is better and more individualized treatments. That includes eliminating overtreatment.

We also need to keep this risk in perspective. Breast cancer is not a scythe hanging over every woman's head. Sometimes it's not even cancer at all. If anything, the recent study should help dial down the fear.

Treating a child's cancer does
not constitute abuse

In 2014, an eleven-year-old girl was condemned to die. A second girl followed suit. How many more? How does anyone dare to call this a victory?

On November 14, 2014, Ontario Court Justice Gethin Edward rejected the pleas of McMaster Children's Hospital to compel child welfare authorities to intervene and force J.J., a member of the Six Nations of the Grand River community who was suffering from leukemia, to resume chemotherapy. Without the treatment, the hospital argued, she had no chance of survival; with chemo, she had a good chance of being cured. The judge ruled that, because of her indigenous status, J.J.'s mother, D.H., has a constitutional right to refuse chemotherapy and "pursue traditional medicine" on the child's behalf. (The family cannot be identified because of a publication ban.)

This is being hailed as a precedent-setting decision for First Nations. It may be a legal victory of sorts, an affirmation and expansion of Section 35 of the Charter of Rights and Freedoms, which guarantees indigenous rights, but it's a hollow one if a child will suffer and die. What we should retain from this case—a case that never should have ended up in court—is that everyone failed to protect a child in need and, by extension, we have failed every child. (Another eerily similar case unfolded at the same time, that of eleven-year-old Makayla Sault of Mississaugas of the New Credit First Nation, but in the court of social media. Diagnosed with acute lymphoblastic leukemia (ALL) in January 2014, she underwent eleven weeks of chemotherapy before she and her parents decided to discontinue treatment. The McMaster Children's Hospital threatened to get a court order to oblige treatment but backed down after an angry response from indigenous leaders. Makayla was treated with traditional medicines as well as at the controversial Hippocrates Health Institute, a "holistic healing centre" in

Florida. She died in January 2015, and her parents said chemotherapy was to blame because it weakened her body.)

J.J. was also diagnosed with ALL. In August 2014, she began treatment and underwent ten days of the planned thirty-two-day course of chemotherapy before her parents rejected the "Western paradigm of medicine" and declared chemo to be poison. Indeed, chemotherapy is poison—poison that kills cancer cells. It's horrible for every child, indigenous or otherwise. It looks as though the hospital did not adequately assuage the parents' fears and could have been more culturally sensitive. When it sought to force the girl back into treatment by legal means, it set up an adversarial relationship. But say this for McMaster Children's: they put the child first, even though they knew pursuing the case would cause them untold grief. The child welfare agency, Brant Family and Children's Services, failed J.J., too. They decided she was not a "child in need of protection" because she had loving parents, and tried to fob off the decision about forced treatment on others. But a child welfare agency has one job: to protect the welfare of children. Anything else is a dereliction of duty.

The court also failed J.J., and spectacularly. In similar cases, where parents have refused life-saving medical interventions for religious reasons (such as Jehovah's Witnesses refusing blood transfusions) or because they reject mainstream medicine for whatever reason, the courts have been quick to intervene and compel treatment. But in this case, the court decided that the parents' indigenous rights should take precedence over the life, liberty and security of an individual child. A judge's role is often to find the proper balance between conflicting rights; in this case, the scales of justice tipped the wrong way. Worse yet, the court afforded the parents the right to opt for "traditional medicine" without defining that term. In fact, Justice Edward said the details of treatment (such as whether it would actually work) were irrelevant; he essentially gave the parents carte blanche to do as they pleased. That was wrong because a child's life hung in the balance. (One of the more disturbing aspects of this case was that J.J.'s alternative "treatment" had been at the Hippocrates Health Institute, a regime of massage and organic vegetables.)

Mercifully, the case had a happy ending. Instead of appealing the court ruling, the hospital, child welfare authorities and the family reached an amicable agreement that saved face for everyone. J.J. retained her right to refuse treatment, but ultimately opted to undergo chemotherapy again, and traditional medicines were incorporated into her care. Media reports suggest she was in remission and thriving in 2016. Without question, horrible abuses and injustices have been rained upon First Nations and their children in particular—consider the residential schools and the gross overrepresentation of indigenous children in Canada's child-welfare and foster-care systems. But treating children like J J and Makayla for cancer—even though it evokes those horrific images of children being snatched from their parents once again—is not one of those abuses. On the contrary.

If a non-indigenous child had been in the same situation as J.J., she would almost certainly have been treated with chemotherapy. Every child needs to be protected from blatantly unreasonable acts by their parents, even well-intentioned ones. The affirmation of indigenous rights should not condemn children to second-class treatment and death. In fact, these cases should never be in the courts and in the headlines. Wrenching ethical issues like the right of a child to refuse cancer treatment cannot be addressed properly with adversarial legal action; they require mediation, education and compassion.

Ultimately, J.J.'s case (and Makayla's too) was about the shifting culture of medicine in which patients are demanding more of a say in their care. If there is one thing everyone can agree on, it's that these girls' parents wanted the best for them. They saw their children suffering while undergoing chemo and wanted it to stop. Obviously, their fears were not assuaged; they were not convinced that benefits outweighed risks. J.J.'s case has reminded us, too, that medicine is often paternalistic. But if patients and their families want to be empowered, if they want to be judge and jury on care decisions, they must also be more responsible and selfless—especially when the life of a child hangs in the balance.

Evidence, not emotion, needs to guide prostate cancer screening and treatment

Gentlemen of a certain age, take note: the dogma around prostate cancer testing and treatment has changed markedly. It's worth taking a minute to think about why, how and even whether you should be tested. Further, if you do have a diagnosis of prostate cancer, you need to seriously consider whether you should actually be treated at all.

At first blush, those statements may seem like heresy. But a landmark study, published in the New England Journal of Medicine in late 2016, has provided some stark data on the benefits, risks and necessity of treatment for men with low- or medium-risk prostate cancer (meaning they have a Gleason score of between 6 and 7). The uplifting news is that, a decade after diagnosis, 99 percent of men with early prostate cancer are still alive. The sort-of-surprising news is that mortality rates don't really vary depending on type of treatment, or whether a man is treated at all. "There's no hard evidence that treating early disease makes a difference," said Freddie Hamdy, a professor of surgery at the University of Oxford and the study's lead author.

Researchers examined data from 82,000 British men who underwent prostate-specific antigen (PSA) testing. Of that total, 2,700 were diagnosed with prostate cancer and 1,643 agreed to be assigned randomly to one of the three groups: prostate surgery, radiation treatment and active monitoring, meaning they were tested regularly to see whether the cancer had spread. Of the 545 men in the active-monitoring group, 33 developed metastases (spread of cancer) and 8 died; among those who had their prostate removed there were 13 metastases and 5 deaths, and in the radiation group, 16 and 4 respectively. In other words, doing "nothing" (surveillance) resulted in just a slightly higher risk of cancer spreading—6 percent versus 3 percent—but not a statistically significant increase in mortality, at least after ten years.

But the catch is this: those who underwent more aggressive

treatment had a lot more side effects. For example, six months after diagnosis, 46 percent of men who underwent prostate surgery were incontinent and using adult diapers, compared to 4 percent in the active-surveillance group. Similarly, only 12 percent of men who underwent surgery were able to sustain an erection, compared to 22 percent in the radiotherapy group and 46 percent in the active-surveillance group. Half the men in the active-monitoring group eventually underwent surgery or radiation but, in the interim, they had better quality of life.

This sort of analysis is important because about 24,000 men are diagnosed with prostate cancer each year in Canada. While everyone wants to be cured, they do not always think of the price to be paid, such as incontinence, impotence and depression. The good news is that, in Canada, active surveillance is already the norm for more than half of patients with localized prostate cancer. But according to research by the Canadian Partnership Against Cancer, rates vary a lot around the country, so more work needs to be done.

The other element of this story is the effectiveness and appropriateness of screening. Prostate-specific antigen testing is one of the most controversial issues in the cancer field. The Canadian Task Force on Preventive Health Care says PSA screening should not be done because it does more harm than good. Large, long-term studies in Europe show that PSA screening reduces cancer mortality by less than 1 percent. Put another way, to prevent one death from prostate cancer, 1,055 men would need to be screened and thirty-seven cancers detected.

Furthermore, for every man who benefits from PSA testing, 27 are harmed by unnecessary treatment—complications such as impotence, incontinence and higher risk of heart disease and osteoporosis (because many men get a hormonal treatment that deprives their body of androgens). Elevated PSA levels trigger biopsies and often lead to a cascade of overtreatment. (To be clear, the PSA test is an excellent tool for monitoring patients who have cancer and are undergoing treatment. The debate revolves around its usefulness as a diagnostic tool. It generates a lot of false positives because PSA levels can shoot up for reasons other than the presence of cancer.)

Prostate cancer kills 4,100 Canadian men a year, but it's not by doing more and earlier testing and more aggressive treatment that we will necessarily reduce that number. Prostate cancer can, in some instances, be extremely aggressive and kill quickly. But by and large, it is slow-growing—a cancer you die with rather than from. That's a hard message to digest, and deliver. What we really need is a test that shows whether prostate cancer, once detected, will prove aggressive and deadly or not, and we don't have that.

The problem is that every man is convinced he is the man who is going to die. No one believes he could be harmed rather than helped by treatment. Years of evidence tells a very different story: the reality is we have imperfect tests and imperfect treatments. More than anything, the latest research provides a welcome reminder that, despite the fear the C-word strikes in our hearts, having a bit of cancer in your body is not necessarily an emergency. Screening is going to give you information that may not be particularly helpful. If you do get a prostate-cancer diagnosis, there is no rush to receive treatment and many reasons to ponder the pros and cons while continuing to live your life to the fullest.

CHAPTER 12

Infectious Disease

What ever happened to SARS?

In late 2002 and early 2003, four letters, s-a-r-s, struck panic in the hearts of the public, politicians and public-health officials. SARS, of course, stands for severe acute respiratory syndrome. When reports of a "fatal flu" emerged from China in late 2002, immediate fears arose that a new pathogen could spread rapidly around the globe. SARS soon dominated the headlines, especially in Canada, one of the hotbeds of the epidemic, and panic spread quickly. In the end, SARS turned out to be relatively mild as infectious diseases go, with a total of 8,096 cases and 774 deaths worldwide. Canada registered 251 cases and 43 deaths; all but a handful of cases occurred in hospitals, making SARS a hospital-acquired infection that posed little risk to the general public. It was, however, economically devastating: the Asian economy took a US$18 billion hit, and the Canadian economy lost C$1.5 billion in 2003, most of it because tourism and travel to affected countries dried up. By July 2003, the World Health Organization declared the outbreak over. Since then, there have been only nine cases, all of them in laboratories doing research on the coronavirus.

So what did we learn? The answer to that question can be found primarily in the thorough report of the eleven-member National Advisory Committee on SARS and Public Health, chaired by Dr. David Naylor and released in October 2003. The committee's report made it clear that Canada's public-health system was ill-prepared to deal with an infectious disease threat. The system had too little money, too few health professionals, a lack of laboratory capacity, inadequate disease surveillance, weak links to the medical system, an overabundance of turf wars and an utter lack of co-ordination. When Naylor began his work, he could not even determine how much was actually spent on public health. The best estimate was no more than $2.8 billion, or less than 2.5 percent of health-care spending. It was also clear that despite the carnage, Canada got off relatively easy because SARS was not very virulent. If the new pathogen had, for example, been a pandemic strain of the flu, the outcome would have been far more dire.

The committee called for $700 million a year in new money, the creation of a Canadian public health agency at arm's length from government, and for a chief public-health officer. Among the committee's seventy-five recommendations were the creation of a national network of communicable disease experts, a national immunization strategy, beefing up the laboratory system and dealing with a critical shortage of public-health nurses and physicians. Those in health circles expressed unprecedented unanimity that Naylor's prescription was the right one, an articulate blueprint for rebuilding the system.

And, for once, governments acted swiftly and decisively on a report's recommendations—considering that fast and thorough are relative terms in the political world. There were redundant rounds of task forces and discussion papers, and the investments weren't what they should have been. In its 2004 budget, the Liberal government bragged that it was spending $1 billion on public health. Yet funding for the new public-health agency, $404 million, was reallocated from within Health Canada; money for a vaccine strategy, $300 million, was to be spread over three years; money for labs and surveillance, only $165 million, was to be spread over two years; and only $100 million each would be allocated for information systems and front-line personnel. It was a far cry from $700 million annually in new money that the Naylor report called for, though Carolyn Bennett, the minister of state for public health, insisted the measures were an "initial investment, a down payment." Sadly, the Public Health Agency of Canada itself also did not measure up to what the doctor ordered. While Naylor had said independence was primordial, the agency would operate "within the Health Canada portfolio." In the end, the chief public health officer was made to report to the minister of health instead of directly to Parliament.

But the most troubling development was the fierce lobbying going on over the location of the new agency's headquarters, with at least five cities vying for bragging rights. (In the end, PHAC ended up in Ottawa, but the National Microbiology Laboratory was built in Winnipeg.) The squabbling was sadly reminiscent of the turf wars that took place during the SARS outbreak, when competing agencies fought over who would be in the media spotlight and researchers bickered about who owned data. It was an approach to public health that Naylor called an "international embarrassment."

Relatively speaking, Canada's response to SARS was no worse, or better, than global agencies like the WHO. An underfunded public-health system managed to wrestle a new pathogen to the ground in record time. In its 2006 report, *SARS: How a Global Epidemic Was Stopped*, the WHO conceded that communications was the biggest failing. The language used, like "global emergency," fuelled panic. And in the end, success in corralling SARS was due to nineteenth-century-style public-health measures like contact tracing, quarantine and infection control. "None of the modern technical tools had an important role to play in control of SARS," the WHO concluded, except the Internet.

SARS was the first global outbreak where data were available in real time and scientists, clinicians and public-health officials worked together on several continents to identify the coronavirus and its source (the Chinese horseshoe bat), trade clinical notes and develop treatments in record time. They learned how to do surveillance, data collection and research and, ultimately, how to communicate with the public in the emerging social-media world. That served us well when a real threat, the pandemic H1N1 influenza, came along in 2009. In short, SARS exposed same gaping holes in public health and gave us an opportunity to patch them up.

Why panic over H1N1 is not the answer

The deaths of two young, previously healthy children in 2009 were bound to terrify families and to ramp up the fear related to H1N1 influenza several notches. Many parents wondered, should we keep our kids home from school, should we keep them away from hockey practice and gymnastics, or should we—horror of horrors—put the kibosh on Halloween? The answer to those questions was no—but an equivocal no. That didn't mean there was no risk, of course. The chances of contracting H1N1 were relatively high, and it was estimated that, by the time all was said and done, as many as one in three Canadians could be afflicted by the disease. Still, that was and remains only slightly higher than seasonal flu. (On average, approximately 12,500 people are hospitalized with severe flu symptoms and 3,500 die annually, but those numbers can vary a lot based on the severity of the circulating strains.)

While H1N1 flu was unpleasant, only a fraction of the infected became so sick that they required hospitalization, and fewer still died. But because the denominator was so large, a lot of severely ill people ended up in intensive care, particularly during flu season, and thousands died. While H1N1 was a pandemic strain, it was no more deadly than a "regular" strain and H1N1 has now become a common circulating strain of the flu that continues to sicken and kill. Statistics, of course, are abstract. The deaths of those two children—their stories and photos splashed across the front page of newspapers and on TV newscasts—were painfully and frighteningly real. The difficulty is putting this risk in context so it too is meaningful.

In twenty-first-century Canada, risk is a largely unfamiliar concept. In a country of thirty-six million people that has nearly 400,000 births annually, fewer than 800 children aged one through fourteen die each year. (Another 1,200 or so under the age of one die, most of congenital abnormalities.) In Canada, the greatest danger to children is falls and motor vehicle collisions. Deaths from infectious disease are remarkably few, in large part due to vaccination. Yet the H1N1 vaccine is hard to come by, even for high-priority groups such as children. And while mass immunization campaigns are rolled out across the nation, the lines are frustratingly long.

The correct answer to the question, "What should parents do?" was this: "Without hesitating, they should bite the bullet and get their children vaccinated. Pack a book, load a new game and some music on your iPhone and get in line. While you're waiting, relish the thought that we live in a country where one of the greatest threats to our children is a bug with a relatively small risk. And don't forget that the risks of the vaccine itself are vanishingly small. Paradoxically, the lineups for the vaccine are creating huge gatherings, something that should be avoided during an outbreak of disease. But this risk too has to be kept in context."

The best and most reasoned information on the matter came from the US Centers for Disease Control and Prevention, which in 2010 published a document titled *Guidance for State and Local Public Health Officials and School Administrators for School (K-12) Responses to Influenza*. The guidelines stated, essentially, that closing schools is unnecessary, except in circumstances with huge numbers of infected students and staff. (Similar reasoning applies to other community activities such as sports and trick-or-treating.) The CDC report suggested that individual children (and adults) should stay home if sick to avoid infecting others. But closing schools only creates alternate gathering places, such as malls and makeshift daycares. The CDC also said that when children (and adults) are out and about, they should practise hand hygiene and etiquette to minimize the spread of germs. Only in rare instances should activities be cancelled. In other words, life can and should go on during flu season. Isolation and quarantine are not very effective public-health measures on a large scale. They don't substantially reduce the risk of the spread of disease and they greatly increase panic and fear.

In any case, what is risk? The dictionary definition is "the possibility of suffering harm or loss: danger." A more modern and timely definition comes from risk-management guru Peter Sandman, a former professor at Rutgers University and the creator of the formula "Risk = Hazard + Outrage." We know, in a mathematical way, the risk of H1N1 influenza: low but still significant. What is more difficult to measure is outrage, or fear.

When children die, fear rises in an exponential manner. If nothing else, the tragic deaths of Evan Frustaglio, thirteen, of Toronto, and Vanetia Warner, ten, of Cornwall, Ontario, should have shaken Canadians out of their complacency. But the masses should not hurtle to the other extreme, panic. Between complacency and panic is a vast territory—one we should occupy actively, by working, by going to school and, yes, by trick-or-treating.

—————⋀⋁—————

Prevention holds the ultimate key to stemming the AIDS epidemic

I n the summer of 1854, London, England, experienced a cholera epidemic. At the time, it was believed that the disease was transmitted through miasma—bad air. Dr. John Snow wasn't so sure. So he plotted cholera deaths on a map and interviewed family members of the deceased. The evidence showed all had drunk from the Broad Street pump, a local water supply. Snow famously removed the handle from the pump and stopped the epidemic in its tracks, decades before scientists confirmed that cholera is caused by a water-borne bacterium. The pioneering work became the basis of the science of epidemiology and the foundation of the modern public-health movement.

Acquired immune deficiency syndrome, or AIDS, has been the greatest challenge ever posed to public health—perhaps to humanity itself—but Snow's actions can still inform and guide modern science. According to the World Health Organization, at the end of 2015 over seventy-eight million people had been infected with the human immunodeficiency virus (HIV), and over thirty-five million deaths had been reported. Plotting and mapping the disease tells us that the pandemic, which exploded in the early 1980s, is in fact a series of distinct yet intertwined epidemics affecting groups as diverse as men who have sex with men, blood transfusion recipients and hemophiliacs, intravenous drug users and migrant workers who use the services of sex workers. There are also related geographic outbreaks beginning in San Francisco, then Haiti, sub-Saharan Africa and the former Soviet Union, plus pockets of China and India.

Modern epidemiology, bolstered with technology, allows us to know not only where people were infected with HIV-AIDS, but how and when. This, in turn, gives us valuable information on where we should focus prevention efforts. In Canada, the disease is spreading among intravenous drug users and indigenous people; in China, in recipients of blood transfusions; in India, among long-distance truck drivers who frequent sex workers; in sub-Saharan Africa, in heterosexual women whose partners are having unprotected sex with multiple partners.

Individual behavioural patterns remain the principal reason for the spread of HIV-AIDS. But social, cultural and economic factors also influence behaviour. Like all other health issues, socio-economic determinants of health play a key role in the spread of the disease and how people protect themselves, or not: they need clean water, food, housing, income and legal protections to have even a fighting chance. Women whose economic security and identity depend on having children will not use condoms; men who are incarcerated will often have sex with other men; a certain percentage of the population will turn to sex workers regardless of the risks; a certain level of drug use exists in all societies in spite of legal prohibitions; and teenaged and premarital sex is going to happen regardless of parents' wishes.

The role of public health is not to pass judgment or be moralistic. It is to minimize harm. Public-health officials cannot be guided by religious tenets, cultural taboos or individual enthusiasm or disdain for practices and programs. They have to be guided by science, by the best available evidence of what minimizes risk and reduces harm. There is no magic bullet. But there is still much that can be done to slow the spread of disease. Good, solid research shows that making condoms available reduces the risk of infection with HIV-AIDS—that is true for heterosexuals and homosexuals, young and old, prisoners and prostitutes. A growing body of evidence suggests that circumcision reduces the risk of transmission. Research shows that needle exchange and safe-injection sites reduce transmission of disease in intravenous drug users. Science tells us that teaching the benefits of abstinence as part of a detailed sex-education program is helpful in reducing unsafe sex, but that abstinence-only education is not.

While much has been said and written about the need—the moral obligation, even—to provide treatment to everyone suffering from HIV-AIDS, regardless of where they live, the same logic should apply to prevention programs. Yet worldwide, fewer than half of people at risk of contracting the disease have any access to prevention measures, even cheap, effective measures such as condom distribution. That is a level of negligence bordering on criminal.

The case for prevention can be made in economic as well as scientific terms. One of the most promising developments is that the global public-health community is embracing the "treatment as prevention" philosophy. If infected people are treated with antiretroviral drugs, the chances of them spreading the disease drop to almost zero, in addition to keeping them healthy and economically productive. Today, 17 million of the 36.7 million people infected with HIV-AIDS around the world are on treatment. Getting everyone who can benefit on treatment is not easy or cheap—even with rock-bottom prices that are offered in the developing world (about US$200 for drugs and another $200 annually for related health care such as testing and checkups). The United Nations, in June 2016, set a bold goal of eliminating new HIV infections by 2030. Practically, that means the number of new infections annually needs to drop from 2.1 million today to below 500,000 by 2020, and then to close to zero by 2030. To get there, UNAIDS has an action planned dubbed "90-90-90." That means taking the following measures:

- Ensuring that 90 percent of the infected are tested and diagnosed; currently, that number is about 57 percent.
- Getting 90 percent of those who are diagnosed onto treatment with antiretroviral drugs; that number is currently 46 percent.
- Aiming to have at least 90 percent of those infected attain

an undetectable level of virus in their bodies (essentially a functional cure); currently, those rates range from 40 to 80 percent in various countries but sit at only 38 percent overall.

That's only phase one. The hard part is completing the final 10-10-10, those who are hardest to reach and who are fuelling the epidemic: vulnerable and marginalized populations like sex workers, intravenous drug users, prisoners, transgender people, indigenous people, refugees and adolescent girls. But even if by some miracle HIV transmission is eliminated by 2030, millions of people will still be living with HIV, and they will be around for a generation and likely more.

It does not matter how much good science we have unless we implement the findings, unless we have the courage and foresight to act. We have done the mapping. We know the source and the impact of HIV-AIDS and a whole lot about how to mitigate the galloping spread of the epidemic. For more than thirty-five years, we've been "removing the handles" in the manner of John Snow and trying to stem the carnage. But the work is far from done.

With AIDS, we've come a long way ... maybe

C anada has hosted the International AIDS Conference more often than any other country—Montreal in 1989, Vancouver in 1996 and Toronto in 2006. What started as a purely scientific meeting in 1985, the International AIDS Conference was held in response to the discovery of the human immunodeficiency virus when the epidemic of HIV-AIDS was in its infancy. But as the number of infections soared and people with HIV-AIDS (particularly, in the early years, gay men) became increasingly angry and militant, it became an important political and social forum as well.

Given how politically loaded the choice of venue is, there is a tacit recognition here that Canada is not only home to an impressive number of world-class HIV-AIDS researchers but also that this country is perceived as a model of tolerance and social justice. HIV-AIDS, after all, is a disease that has disproportionately affected the marginalized of society—gay men, intravenous drug users, sex workers, indigenous people, street youth, the sick (notably transfusion recipients) and the poor and powerless of society (particularly girls and women in the developing world). But does Canada deserve this reputation as both a social and scientific leader in HIV-AIDS?

The medical treatment of people with HIV-AIDS is certainly good, with specialized treatment centres like Clinique médicale l'Actuel in Montreal, and the clinics at St. Michael's Hospital in Toronto and St. Paul's Hospital in Vancouver. We have top-notch researchers such as Julio Montaner of the BC Centre for Excellence in HIV/AIDS in Vancouver and Mark Wainberg of McGill University in Montreal. Canada also leads the way in providing so-called drug cocktails, combinations of drugs that have markedly extended the lifespan of people with the disease. But a 2007 study commissioned by the Public Health Agency of Canada showed that patients still face many challenges out there. The research, conducted by Environics Research Group, was based on focus groups of people living with HIV-AIDS. It showed that, three decades into the epidemic, stigma and discrimination are still pervasive.

In the early days of the virus, the fear was palpable. Gay men became pariahs. They were evicted from their apartments and some lost their jobs. People feared they could catch this deadly "plague" from toilet seats in public places. Those attitudes and irrational fears lingered for a long time. In October 1988, when social activism surrounding HIV-AIDS was really taking off, *The Globe and Mail* ran a story about a gay man admitted to a Toronto hospital for treatment of a urinary tract infection. He was not HIV-positive, but health workers posted a large pink sign over his bed warning that he posed a "high risk of contamination." Some staff refused to touch him.

Today, because of HIV-AIDS, all hospitals have adopted "universal precautions," meaning that all patients are treated as if they might have an infectious disease, so staff wear gloves and dispose of needles and other sharp objects in a prescribed manner. But according to the focus groups, the place where people with HIV-AIDS still feel the sting of discrimination most is in the health-care system. When HIV-positive patients deal with specialized clinics, they have nothing but praise for the care. It is when they enter the mainstream system for the treatment of everyday ills—broken bones, a toothache, a heart attack, minor surgery—that the negative experiences occur. For many years, they were refused elective procedures and surgeries—from dental appointments on up—on the wrong-headed assumption that they posed a risk to health professionals and that other patients are more deserving because those with HIV-AIDS have a death sentence. With the adoption of universal precautions, the risks to health-care providers, which were never high in the first place, are virtually non-existent. And, as knowledge of HIV-AIDS has grown, stigma has faded a lot. But there are still challenges.

One of the hottest debates in medico-ethical circles in recent years has revolved around transplantation in people with HIV-AIDS. Drug cocktails have extended the life expectancy of sufferers so markedly that they are now developing the same chronic conditions as the HIV-negative population. They need kidney, liver and heart transplants just like others. The blanket exclusion of HIV-positive patients from transplant lists—until quite recently, the norm—has disappeared, but the bar for eligibility is still set a little higher.

Because of the way they are treated, one of the issues people with HIV-AIDS struggle with is disclosure—does one disclose one's status and risk discrimination and stigmatization, or not disclose and worry about being discovered? In some cases, such as transplantation, there are sound medical and ethical reasons to disclose. But in most everyday health-care situations, HIV status is irrelevant.

What comes through clearly from the focus groups is the message that people with HIV-AIDS long for the day when their status is irrelevant and being HIV-positive does not affect the way they are perceived or cared for in any way. What they want, and what they deserve, is to be treated like Joe Average—with apologies to Vancouver artist and

AIDS activist Joe Average. That would indeed make Canada a model of tolerance and social justice. It would also make for a better health-care system for everyone.

—√ᴸ—

People with AIDS face a tyrant
called indifference

Like most big medical conferences, the International AIDS Conference in Vienna, Austria, in 2010 was held in a giant, soulless convention centre. But with its odd mix of scientists, clinicians, politicians, humanitarian groups, social activists, rock stars and business moguls, it was not your typical medical meeting. Beyond the dry scientific presentations and weighty research abstracts was a parallel stream of street theatre in the form of die-ins, political speeches, condom distribution, trashing of exhibitor booths and well-orchestrated multilingual protests. A much-anticipated march through the streets of the host city served to underscore the conference's theme and provided valuable video and photos for media outlets tired of dour images of talking heads at a podium.

At the AIDS Conference in Durban, South Africa, back in 2000, the protest was electrifying. Activists embraced the theme "Breaking the Silence" with an impressive display of vuvuzelas, whistles, songs and chants. That protest, as much as the conference itself, served as a catalyst for the movement to get cheap antiretroviral drugs to those who were desperately in need in developing countries. (Today, almost half of the world's AIDS sufferers are receiving treatment.)

In Vienna, the protest was more subdued but no less memorable. That is because the march, which shared the meeting's theme "Rights Here, Rights Now," culminated in Heldenplatz (Heroes' Square). The choice was deliberate and the symbolism powerful. Heldenplatz is where Adolf Hitler gave one of his more infamous speeches, announcing the Anschluss—literally "link-up," the euphemism used to describe the forced annexation of Austria, the first step in the expansion of Germany that would eventually trigger the Second World War. The ornate Parliament, where the Nazi banner was once displayed, was adorned with a giant red ribbon, the symbol of solidarity with those who are HIV-positive. Where Austrians once stood listening to the hateful words of a tyrant espousing racial purity and world domination, there gathered one of the most diverse crowds imaginable, giving voice to the voiceless.

The delegates' message was delivered on signs, in chants and in song, but principally by their presence. There were people who were HIV-positive and HIV-negative, black and white (and every shade in between), African and European, gay and straight and bi, male and female and transgender, sex workers and scientists, prisoners and politicians, IV drug users and drug company reps, Jews and Gentiles. Diverse but with a single message: human rights are universal.

On the Heldenplatz, the juxtaposition of old and new, of history and future challenges, was thought-provoking. Bullets and bombs once claimed a generation, while today it is a microscopic virus. Tyranny once came in human form—Adolf Hitler. Today it is more banal—a lack of humanity, 36.7 million people in the world living with HIV-AIDS and 2.1 million new infections annually, not to mention 1.1 million AIDS-related deaths (statistics from the end of 2015).

HIV-AIDS is a treatable and preventable condition—like most other infectious diseases. Yet half of those who would benefit from treatment are not getting it, and prevention programs are not nearly as extensive as they should be. Despite the lack of a vaccine, science has made tremendous gains in the battle against HIV-AIDS. But progress on the ground has been stalled by our lack of dedication to human rights. The persecution of high-risk groups such as homosexual men and intravenous drug users, coupled with a glaring lack of gender equality in much of the world, continues to fuel the global epidemic.

Human rights are essential to good health. Treating people better leads to better treatment. Students of history will know that the Anschluss was a gross violation of the Treaty of Versailles, but the Allies responded with little more than a shrug. Hitler was emboldened and his outrages would escalate into the Holocaust. The tyrant slaughtered six million members of minority groups—primarily Jews, but also gays, gypsies and the mentally and physically disabled.

While some may bristle at the analogy, HIV-AIDS is a public-health holocaust. The disease has arguably had a greater impact on Africa than slavery. Like all effective tyrants, it targets the vulnerable—in this case Africans, gays, indigenous peoples, drug users. The silence to their plight is sometimes deafening; rich Western countries like Canada have reacted with grand words but far less grand gestures. These days the claim is that the budget shortfall has left them unable to do more to stem the pandemic, but it is a matter of priorities. As Dr. Julio Montaner, former president of the International AIDS Society, said, "When there is a Wall Street emergency or an oil spill, billions upon billions of dollars are quickly mobilized. When there is a need for a rapid response to the global health crisis of HIV-AIDS, people's health deserves a similar response, and yet we cannot find it."

Since the beginning of the pandemic, approximately seventy-eight million people have been infected with HIV, and thirty-seven million have died of AIDS. Despite a massive public-health response and impressive scientific progress, there are still 240 new infections every hour. Far too many people have been, and continue to be, victims of a tyrant called indifference.

—╱╲—

Breathing life into the century-old battle against tuberculosis

In the two weeks leading up to Christmas, 1908, the *Globe* (before it merged with *The Mail and Empire*) helped launch a historic campaign to stamp out tuberculosis, the public-health scourge of the times. It did so by aggressively promoting Christmas Seals—festive stamps whose proceeds went to charity. At the time, the stamps sold at ten for a penny, yet the campaign raised almost $10,000 for the Muskoka Free Hospital for Consumptives.

While TB is now a rarity in Canada—with the exception of remote indigenous communities, where the disease remains a potent symbol of neglect—Christmas Seals remain. (Worldwide, the ancient killer, dubbed the "White Death," is still a scourge, infecting an estimated 10.4 million people and killing 1.8 million in 2015. It always was, and remains, a disease of poverty.) You can still buy the colourful stamps and you can also order them online, available at www.lung.ca. That a charitable campaign is still going strong after more than a century is impressive in itself, but the story of Christmas Seals is, in many ways, a microcosm of the history of health care in Canada.

In 1908, tuberculosis was the number-one killer in this country. About ten thousand people a year died of TB. Yet only fifty treatment beds were available. In the days before medicare, health care was largely unaffordable. This was especially true for an illness such as TB, whose only treatment was bed rest and fresh air. Only the wealthy could afford to be cared for in a rural sanatorium for months, or even years. Back then, Canada had no department of health and only bare-bones public-health measures. The money raised by the Canadian Association for the Prevention of Consumption and Other Forms of Tuberculosis (now the Canadian Lung Association) through the sale of Christmas Seals helped build a public-health infrastructure and create a consumer-health movement. Christmas Seals paid for the country's first mass public-health campaigns—billboards and parade floats that educated the public about tuberculosis prevention. (The *Globe* was particularly enthusiastic about anti-spitting measures.) The monies raised were also used to train doctors and nurses to provide public-health education, something that was previously unheard of. And, of course, money went to research.

Christmas Seals had their origins in Denmark, where postman Einar Holboell, while sorting piles of Christmas mail late one night, glanced out the window to see two hungry waifs freezing in the snow. "What if every Christmas letter or parcel carried an extra stamp and the money went to desperate children?" he wondered. The King of

Denmark liked the idea, so Christmas Seals were born in 1904. Danes purchased a staggering four million Christmas Seals, and two hospitals for children with TB were built.

The idea was imported to Canada a few years later, and since then has raised, conservatively, more than $350 million. That's a lot of stamps. In 1908, Christmas Seals were sold only in Toronto, Hamilton and Winnipeg, but other centres gradually jumped on board, and in the late 1920s the campaign went national. The power of the message became evident in 1929, when the Saskatchewan government promised free TB treatment for all. This bold gesture laid the foundations for the creation of medicare three decades later.

As research and treatment expanded, it became obvious that early diagnosis was the key to controlling the spread of tuberculosis. The Canadian Tuberculosis Association launched massive X-ray campaigns, sending mobile clinics across the country. By 1938, Canada had sixty-one TB sanatoriums with almost nine thousand beds. When soldiers came home from the Second World War, many had TB, causing a massive spike in the disease. By 1953, there were nineteen thousand TB treatment beds nationwide.

But the 1950s also saw the first dramatic breakthrough with the advent of antibiotics to treat TB. The sanatoriums began to empty and to be transformed into hospitals in Canada's burgeoning health-care system. The advent of antibiotics marked a dramatic shift in the health of the population because they provided a potent weapon against bacterial infections like tuberculosis. Today, TB is not only treatable, it is curable at very little cost, though the six-month regimen of antibiotics can be onerous.

While TB was under control, Christmas Seals became more popular than ever. Throughout the 1960s and 1970s, massive mail campaigns were held, promoted by celebrities such as figure skater Toller Cranston and musicians Oscar Peterson and Murray McLauchlan. The decline of the use of snail mail in favour of e-mail and the virtual disappearance of TB have led to a gradual decline in sales of Christmas Seals. Yet the need has not diminished. The relative popularity of smoking has ensured that lung disease remains. So has the increase in allergies and asthma.

Infectious diseases have been, from time immemorial, the world's biggest killers. Tuberculosis alone killed more people than all wars and famines combined. But as deaths from infectious disease fell, deaths from chronic illnesses such as heart disease, stroke, cancer and lung disease rose. Today, they are by far the biggest killers. Chronic obstructive pulmonary disease, a degenerative and debilitating lung condition, is today the country's third-biggest killer, and lung cancer is the biggest cancer killer. While TB killed one Canadian an hour in 1908, COPD killed more than one Canadian an hour in 2015. Although it doesn't have the high profile of cancer or cardiovascular disease, lung disease is the third-leading killer of Canadians—and the only one of the three that is on the rise.

Over a century after Christmas Seals' beginnings, funds raised still go to prevention and research into a multitude of crippling respiratory diseases. But despite much progress, nothing has truly been stamped out. We still can't breathe easy.

—╶╱╲╶—

No outbreak of Ebola, but an outbreak of anxiety

There was never an outbreak of Ebola in North America. But as the number of media stories about the worrisome spread of the disease in West Africa multiplied, there was an outbreak of anxiety—one that, at times, seemed to be veering toward hysteria. So, who was to blame for this sorry state of affairs? And what is the solution? Let's start with the latter.

Every expert in risk communication will tell you that the worst thing you can do when people are worried is tell them not to panic. Rather, you need to provide information. Facts are the antidote to fear. So here are the facts of Ebola: since the outbreak began in West Africa in December 2013, there have been 28,616 cases and 11,310 deaths, almost all of them in Liberia, Sierra Leone and Guinea. Nigeria, Mali and Senegal had small, related outbreaks, but they were quashed. A couple of dozen cases were treated abroad, notably in Spain, Britain and the United States. The World Health Organization declared the "public health emergency of international concern" related to Ebola to be over in March 2016.

The United States, where the media coverage was most intense and sometimes over the top, had a grand total of eight Ebola cases—six of whom were infected in West Africa and airlifted home for care, and two nurses who contracted the disease while caring for these patients. There was one death—Liberian Thomas Eric Duncan, who was already gravely ill when he arrived at a Dallas hospital. In Canada, there were a few false alarms but no Ebola patients.

Not a single person was infected in a plane, train, automobile or other public place. This is not surprising, because the Ebola virus is not airborne; the risk comes from being exposed to the bodily fluids (blood, vomit, etc.) of someone who is infected. The only people really at risk are those caring for the sick and dying, principally nurses, physicians and loved ones and, even there, the risk is low because hospitals have been practising universal precautions since AIDS emerged as a blood-borne threat. The two infected US nurses both cared for Duncan before they knew he had Ebola; they were the only cases of domestic transmission. The health workers infected in West Africa were at much higher risk because they often have to work in crude conditions, lacking even basic protective equipment like masks and gloves.

So, given the negligible risk in the United States and Canada, why did Ebola cause so much anxiety? Some of it has to do with human nature: we tend to fear new and unusual threats more than common ones, no matter how theoretical. Ebola is a killer bug that comes from deepest, darkest Africa, so it's scary. As Dan Gardner wrote in the fabulous book *Risk: The Science and Politics of Fear* (Emblem, 2009), "So much of what we think and do about risk does not make sense." In other words, a certain amount of irrational fear is to be expected. But merchants of fear—politicians, corporations, activists and media— exploit and magnify that irrational fear. And that is how you get the hysteria we saw in 2014—at least in the virtual world. (Evidence that the general public was actually fearful and panicking about Ebola is non-existent. But there was plenty of angst.)

Of course, the media get the lion's share of blame for fear mongering. It is easy to blame the 24/7 news cycle and the proliferation of social media for all the woes of the world. But the media are not a big amorphous blob with a singular narrative. If you want detailed, sublime stories on Ebola, you can find them; you can also find a lot of conspiracy theories, or you can just read the headlines. The worst headline-generating excesses were committed by US politicians, who cranked up the Ebola rhetoric for partisan purposes. But Ebola is an issue that can and should be handled by public-health officials. In general, they have done so fairly well. Most of the mistakes were made at an institutional level, notably at the Dallas hospital where poor infection-control training of health-care workers resulted in two nurses becoming infected.

What public-health officials need to do is continue preparing for worst-case scenarios while providing the public with factual information. These outbreaks—SARS, H1N1 and now Ebola—follow a predictable pattern: at the outset, little information is available and speculation is rampant, and that generates worry; then follows a measure of panic and even hysteria, most of it driven by those exploiting the fear; then the reality sets in and we get around to writing about the fact that panic is unwarranted. The final stage is the realization that once again there were excesses, and some lessons to be learned, especially about how we measure and communicate risk. That can't come soon enough.

CHAPTER 13

Lifestyles

A slow burn will win the
anti-smoking race

Tobacco is a bizarre consumer product. If it were introduced today as a hot new item, it would never be approved by regulatory authorities. Yet through the vagaries of history, it is available for sale and continues to sell remarkably well. About thirty billion cigarettes are sold each year in Canada. Tobacco is still a $1.5-billion-a-year industry. It is a drug that is widely available over the counter even though it has no demonstrable benefits. Tobacco has many more risks than most other prescription, non-prescription or illicit drugs. In fact, it kills far more people than all other drugs combined and is one of the only drugs that can kill through secondary exposure.

Yet, for a product that contains many known carcinogens and toxins, laws regulating its production and use are pretty tame. The Tobacco Act regulates advertising, promotion, packaging, ignition propensity and sales to minors and requires manufacturers to produce mountains of reports right down to the precise content of products. However, there is a provision in the federal Hazardous Products Act that prevents the government from outright prohibiting of tobacco products, as it can do with any other chemical concoction sold to consumers.

The Canada Pension Plan, which invests federal pension contributions, and the Caisse de dépôt et placement du Québec, which does the same in Quebec, also have millions of dollars in tobacco stocks, meaning the state is actually investing in the production of cigarettes. This seems anomalous. After all, tobacco is the only legal product for which the government's stated goal is to suppress use entirely rather than promote safe or responsible use, as it does with alcohol, fatty foods and motor vehicles. The pension funds, however, argue that these stocks are part of larger funds and screening them out would be difficult and result in lower returns.

All this raises the question, should tobacco be banned outright? Paradoxically, no, it should not. There are approximately 5.4 million smokers in Canada, and about 80 percent of them are addicted to nicotine. It is an addiction that can be all consuming, and smokers would suffer greatly and unjustly from a ban. Tobacco prohibition would be a bonanza for smugglers and sellers of contraband cigarettes. There would also be no small measure of hypocrisy in suddenly banning the sale of cigarettes and related products. Governments have profited handsomely from the sale of tobacco. For a long time, they tacitly endorsed tobacco use and heavily subsidized its producers. Even today, anti-smoking initiatives focus largely on punishing smokers. They are taxed heavily—including direct taxes on cigarettes and higher insurance rates—and their ability to smoke is increasingly restricted by regulation.

These measures are not inappropriate, but they are insufficient to reduce smoking and unfair to smokers. To date, public-health measures such as taxation, banning advertising, age restrictions, regulating packaging and smoking bans have focused on reducing demand for cigarettes and the attractiveness of smoking. But, as the US Institute of Medicine pointed out in a 2007 report, we have largely failed to address the addictive aspects of tobacco and to constrain manufacturers' ability to woo more smokers. Until we do, we are unlikely to get smoking rates much below the current Canadian levels of 18 percent of adults, let alone eliminate smoking entirely.

The Institute of Medicine, in its report titled *Ending the Tobacco Problem: A Blueprint for the Nation*, said the focus should shift to tobacco manufacturers. Its most intriguing recommendation was that federal health authorities—the US Food and Drug Administration and Health Canada—should have the right to regulate tobacco products like other drugs. The institute suggested that this power be used to regulate the amount of nicotine in cigarettes—that the amount of nicotine released in each cigarette be fully disclosed on the package (as is the active ingredient in all regulated drugs), standardized and gradually diminished over time. This way, smokers can be weaned off the addictive substance, and governments weaned from their addiction to tobacco taxes. The report also called for dramatic increases in health-promotion budgets, suggesting annual per-capita spending of about US$20 on tobacco control.

Currently Canada spends only a fraction of that amount—about C$1 on tobacco control for every $100 it collects in tobacco taxes. The budget for the federal tobacco-control strategy was $45 million in 2016—and the provinces spend roughly the same again. Meanwhile, federal and provincial governments collected roughly $8.3 billion in tobacco taxes, not including the Goods and Services Tax.

Given the continuing popularity of smoking among teenagers (girls in particular), it is clear not nearly enough is being done. There is not enough support, either, for smokers who are trying to quit. Smokers' hotlines are inadequate, just as heroin hotlines would be. The report calls for insurance plans (private and public) to be obliged, by law, to pay for smoking-cessation programs.

The IOM 2007 report contained many recommendations, including the following (those already implemented in large part in Canada are marked with an asterisk):

- Ban smoking in all indoor non-residential spaces.*
- Raise tobacco taxes.*
- Dedicate US$20 per capita to tobacco control.
- Require private and public health plans to cover smoking-cessation aids and programs.
- Ban online sales of tobacco.
- Give the regulator, the US Food and Drug Administration, the power to regulate tobacco products like other drugs.
- Limit tobacco advertising.*

- Require large pictorial warnings of the harmful effects of smoking on packages.*
- Prohibit tobacco companies from using the misleading terms *light* and *mild*.*
- Greatly restrict the type and number of outlets that can sell tobacco products, and require them to display warnings and promote smoking-cessation aids.
- Prohibit tobacco companies from sponsoring events that target youth.*
- Regulate and gradually reduce the nicotine content of cigarettes.

Boldly, the institute suggested that smoking rates could be reduced to the single digits by 2025. But as the blueprint states, this can only be achieved if we continue with existing measures while addressing more directly the addictive aspects of tobacco—by constraining the nicotine in each cigarette and relentlessly supporting smokers in their bid to butt out.

Let's take bolder steps to stamp out smoking

For years, we have been gradually tightening the noose on smokers with public-health measures, such as restricting smoking in the workplace, hiking tobacco taxes, introducing graphic warnings on cigarette packages, ending tobacco-company sponsorship of sporting and artistic events, outlawing advertising, eliminating flavoured products that target children, banishing tobacco products from pharmacies, hiding them out of sight in corner stores and banning smoking in bars, restaurants, patios, parks, beaches and so on.

These measures have been relatively effective. Since 1980, Canada has cut the percentage of women and men who smoke by half. But progress has been slow and gradual. There are still about 5.4 million regular smokers, or 18 percent of adults in Canada. In 2015, more than forty thousand Canadians died of tobacco-related illnesses, principally cardiovascular disease, chronic obstructive pulmonary disease (COPD) and cancer. (And not just lung cancer; smoking is linked to cancers of the esophagus, larynx, mouth, throat, kidney, bladder, liver, pancreas, stomach, cervix, colon and rectum, as well as acute myeloid leukemia.) But tobacco remains a legal product, one that is widely used and quite profitable, despite the fact that it is lethal.

Are Canadians going to content ourselves with quietly encouraging smokers to quit and passively hoping young people will not begin smoking and expecting that the problem will resolve itself somehow, some day in the distant future? Or are we going to set hard targets for the elimination of tobacco? After decades of short-term, largely local measures, it's time to embrace some bold national initiatives. The endgame needs to be clear: to eradicate the use of tobacco products and the diseases they cause in the near future. That means there needs to be hard deadlines, say, 2025 for Canada and 2040 for the rest of the world. (Most countries define being "tobacco free" as having fewer than 5 percent of adults who smoke.)

So how do we get there? There are a number of possible strategies:

- *Prohibition.* Tobacco is a toxic, addictive substance with little or no redeeming value that creates a great health and economic burden. Banning it outright would be justifiable but probably ineffective. We have to bear in mind that governments have both tolerated and profited from tobacco for a long time, and punishing nicotine addicts would be cruel.
- *Tobacco-free generation.* Singapore has a proposal for a line-in-the-sand approach—to bar anyone born after 2000 from buying or consuming tobacco products, with the aim of gradually phasing out its sale and use. A novel idea, but probably difficult to enforce in most countries.
- *Shrinking supply.* You take a base year of tobacco sales, and then reduce supply by 10 percent a year and, in a decade, there is no more tobacco sold. New Zealand is taking this tack, but it can

only work in a country that is relatively isolated and can strictly control imports.

· *A regulated market.* Make the government solely responsible for the marketing and distribution of tobacco (similar to the LCBO monopoly over alcohol in Ontario) then gradually choke off supply. A number of countries have state-run tobacco production and sales—notably China, home to one-third of the world's smokers—but they have little incentive to reduce sales sharply.

· *Prescription-only tobacco.* Make tobacco a controlled substance but allow access to those with an addiction. With this approach, you limit access to new smokers, but don't punish long-time smokers. However, a vigorous black market would likely arise, as with other prescription drugs.

· *Nicotine-reduction legislation.* Strictly regulate the amount of nicotine in cigarettes, and force manufacturers to reduce it over time, so smokers are tapered off their addiction, and tobacco becomes less addictive. The US Food and Drug Administration is considering this approach.

Ultimately, the solution likely will be a combination of some of these measures as well as the more traditional public-health and harm-reduction approaches. In general, much more serious efforts need to be invested in smoking cessation, in helping people who want to quit (which is most of the smoking population) actually quit.

And, of course, new challenges will crop up along the way, such as those involving e-cigarettes. These create a conundrum because they have the potential to eliminate the most damaging aspect of smoking (the smoke and other by-products of combustion are what cause disease and death, not nicotine), but they can also undermine anti-smoking efforts by normalizing the act of smoking (or vaping) anew.

With one billion smokers worldwide and six million smoking-related deaths a year, we cannot underestimate the challenge. Traditional, cautious tobacco-control measures will take forever to have a lasting impact, and deaths will pile up by the millions. The carnage inflicted by smoking has gone on far too long. Surely, the time for half measures has passed. Some urgency is in order in the quest for a tobacco-free world.

——————

The dilemma of e-cigarettes

Rarely has a single product evoked such diametrically opposed views or such passion as e-cigarettes. Anti-smoking activists see the electronic nicotine-delivery systems (the formal name) as another evil concoction of Big Tobacco, a devilish way to create new smokers and undermine hard-fought public-health measures. Proponents of e-cigarettes see them as a means of getting what they desperately want—usually nicotine, and sometimes simply the tactile act of smoking—without the carcinogens in tobacco, and as means of gaining freedom from the increasingly oppressive measures taken against smokers.

E-cigarettes are canisters used to simulate the act of smoking: batteries heat up fluid-filled cartridges that contain water, flavouring agents and often, though not always, nicotine. The act of smoking an e-cigarette is known as *vaping* because you inhale vapours, not smoke.

Health Canada does not approve the sale of e-cigarettes containing nicotine, but this is largely unenforced, and they are widely available. It is also illegal in Canada to make any health claims about e-cigarettes, for example, suggesting they are a smoking-cessation tool. The United States has, to date, taken a hands-off approach, though the US Food and Drug Administration has served notice that it intends to extend its regulatory control of tobacco to e-cigarettes in the near future. Without question, e-cigarettes pose a dilemma for regulators and anti-smoking activists. Devotees—who are an unusually fanatical lot—can trot out amazing anecdotal stories about the power of e-cigarettes and five-pack-a-day smokers who have become healthy vapers. Skeptics feel the arguments are eerily similar to options that have been touted in the past as being "healthier," like "light" cigarettes, cigarellos and chewing tobacco.

Dreams and fears aside, research on e-cigarettes—about their potential harms and potential benefits—is in its infancy. Data on long-term risks and benefits are especially lacking. In other words, the jury is still out, despite the grandiose claims of benefit from proponents and the dire warnings of opponents. In a world with one billion smokers and with smoking killing six million people a year, this is a high-stakes debate. In 2016, the global e-cigarette market surpassed us$6 billion—with more than half of all sales in the us—and the popularity of vaping continues to grow. And everyone is keeping a close eye on China—e-cigarettes were first commercialized in China and introduced in the United States in 2006—because, as it pushes to restrict tobacco, it is touting e-cigarettes as an alternative.

Many anti-smoking activists see e-cigarettes as a Trojan horse, a gateway drug that will attract new users to tobacco and discourage current smokers from quitting. It is not clear how many so-called "dual users" (people who alternate vaping and smoking) exist. Then there is the fear that decades of effort to restrict smoking will be all for naught. At the 2014 People's Choice Awards, for example, vaping was *de rigeur*, to the point where it looked like a product placement for the popular brand Blu. The use of aggressive advertising using recognizable Hollywood stars is reminiscent of the old techniques of Big Tobacco, and public-health officials have pushed back, with most jurisdictions regulating e-cigarettes exactly like cigarettes. (At the 2015 People's Choice Awards, for example, vaping was not visible.)

The point of anti-smoking laws and bylaws is to limit exposure to second-hand smoke, but if vapours are harmless, the argument for restrictions goes up in smoke. So, do e-cigarettes contain toxic chemicals and carcinogens? That is a point of much contention. Some research says yes, some no. Again, in reality a broad range of products is available, with no standards. But e-cigarettes are principally a nicotine-delivery system. Nicotine is addictive—it's what makes people addicted to cigarettes. It's not particularly harmful; it's the by-products of processing and burning tobacco that cause cancer, heart disease, chronic obstructive pulmonary disease and other health woes of smokers. Isn't it preferable to have people addicted to nicotine alone rather than nicotine and a potpourri of toxins? The answer to that loaded question is yes—if you believe in harm reduction.

Most public-health officials strongly favour harm reduction when it comes to "hard" drugs; the supervised injection site Insite, for example, allows intravenous drug users to inject in a controlled setting with clean needles rather than in back alleys with dirty needles. But making that argument for vaping versus smoking doesn't have as much traction. When it comes to tobacco, most public-health officials argue for abstinence and oppose e-cigarettes.

But the sands are constantly shifting. The Lung Association, for example, went from being an outspoken opponent of e-cigarettes to taking the position that they might be a good smoking cessation tool, a way of weaning people off cigarettes. We don't know yet if e-cigarettes are as effective—or as ineffective—as other forms of nicotine replacement therapy.

The other persuasive argument against electronic cigarettes is that they remain an unproven commodity—we shouldn't be rushing headlong to embrace the technology until we know if there are yet-uncovered risks, or if there are better, safer ways to wean smokers off cigarettes. At the risk of sounding like the conclusion of every research study ever published: more research is needed.

In the meantime, though, it seems irrational and counterproductive to ban e-cigarettes in Canada. A more sensible approach would be to regulate and allow nicotine-delivery devices on the market that don't contain carcinogens. In the war on smoking—which is, after all, a battle to improve the health of individuals and society collectively—e-cigarettes are not a panacea, but they are a step in the right direction.

Gen Flab needs our action

The numbers are predictably ugly: Canadians are heavier, wider and weaker than they were a generation ago. According to a 2009 Statistics Canada study, we are packing on the pounds at an alarming rate, and that weight is accumulating primarily around the belly, where it has the most potential to damage our health. The data are noteworthy because researchers went out and weighed, skin-pinched and exercised thousands of Canadians instead of relying on traditional self-reported data (known colloquially as little white lies). The most troubling revelation in the measures was the decline in the fitness of Canadian children and youth between 1981 and 2009.

The numbers tell us that members of Generation Flabby can barely muster a few crunches, they are left breathless by a minute of step-ups, and their average grip strength is barely enough to hang on to a Big Gulp. The Canadian Health Measures Survey was the first phase of a big undertaking (excuse the pun). In the months and years to come, much more research will published—on blood pressure, cholesterol and exposure to metals and chemicals—that will offer even more insight into the health status of Canadians. While the numbers from the second phase of the research have not yet been crunched, early indications are that the trend is upward, especially for weight and adiposity, but that activity levels are also increasing slightly.

The sole job of Statistics Canada—one it does extremely well—is to measure. It has catalogued a duel epidemic of obesity and inactivity, one that we know will have vast consequences for our economy, our health system and various other aspects of life. What we need now is a response: we need action from politicians, policy-makers, community groups and individuals. Yet leadership has been sorely lacking in this area. We simply don't take the issue seriously. Instead, we trot out lame excuses like "Canadians aren't fatter, they're just bigger" and we hide behind rhetorical notions like "people's weight and fitness are personal choices." Well, nobody chooses to be fat, and nobody wants to be unfit. It's unpleasant and it invariably leads to sickness, social limitations and hefty costs.

The blame for our current Fat Nation lies with all of us. We have built an obesogenic society—one that facilitates and encourages inactivity and weight gain at every turn (or, more accurately, at every sit). We have engineered activity out of our daily lives. Everything has a button, from the garage door opener to the TV remote control to the pepper grinder. And so determined are we to see our children succeed that we sit them on their behinds in a classroom seven hours a day and pretend that is a complete education. After hours, there is homework and a bevy of regimented activities, from music lessons to hockey games (kids are active for only about six minutes during an hour-long game). Free time is spent sitting at home in front of the TV, chatting on Facebook, or playing Xbox.

As we grapple for solutions, we too often forget that the solution to inactivity is not exercise (structured, regimented, goal-oriented), and it is not a token gym class or workout crammed into a hectic schedule. Rather, it is making activity an integral part of everyday life. Running, jumping, skipping, tobogganing, playing tag, walking to school, taking the stairs—that's what children need to be healthy, physically and mentally. Adults need this too. We need to make physical activity (and healthy eating) easy, and a seamless part of everyday life, because regimented programs and diets are usually not enough to break ingrained habits.

But in the age of terrorists-around-every-corner, we have developed a strange set of phobias and misplaced priorities. We have a pervasive fear about the safety of our children, so we don't let them walk to school or play in the park or ride their bikes. But we let them sit in front of the TV for five hours eating processed foods. Parents mean well but seem to have lost sight of what really matters. To have money to give their children everything they need and then some, they work themselves to the bone and move to the long-commute suburbs for a "better life." Hence, they have no time to play with their children, no time to cook at home (so take-out and processed food becomes the daily diet) and no time to care for themselves and set examples.

Stranger danger—the idea that a child will be harmed by a stranger—is exceedingly rare. But the danger done to our children's health by modelling unhealthy and unsustainable lifestyles is very real. The Statistics Canada data scream out a sad reality: our children have learned the lessons we have modelled all too well. Twenty-six percent of children aged six to eleven are overweight or obese, and that number rises to 28 percent in teens. Then the inactivity really begins to show. Sixty-one percent of Canadian adults are overweight or obese. And don't forget they didn't have the head start on weight accumulation that their children have.

There are other data, of course, of varying quality, and with slightly different numbers. But the precise numbers don't matter as much as the trend lines. The message is that collective and individual action is required. Failing to act will have dire consequences. Are we prepared—as one researcher said—to mortgage our children's future? If so, choose inaction and inactivity. Otherwise, individually and collectively, we need to recalibrate—get our priorities straight by putting the health of our children at the top. It starts with a little action, some activity and play, glorious play.

Think running's deadly? Well, nobody's counting the La-Z-Boy deaths

In October 2011, a twenty-seven-year-old man died in the Toronto Marathon. The previous week, a thirty-five-year-old man died in the Chicago Marathon. And in September 2011, a thirty-two-year-old man died in the Montreal Marathon. Three high-profile deaths by cardiac arrest in seemingly healthy men during mass-participation events in less than a month. In September 2015, a thirty-one-year-old woman died in the Montreal Marathon, though her death was overshadowed by the dramatic collapse of a forty-six-year-old man, metres from the finish line, who was revived with a defibrillator—all of which was filmed and broadcast. It gives the distinct impression that long-distance running is dangerous and deadly. How long will it be before there are calls to ban marathons or demands that participants undergo mandatory medical testing before they can run?

As tragic as these deaths are, a knee-jerk response to restrict these types of events would be a mistake. The solution, while seemingly counterintuitive, is to encourage a lot more people to lace 'em up and hit the streets. The benefits far outweigh the risks—regardless of the impression you may get from newspaper headlines. Those who think marathons are deadly dangerous are grossly misinformed: they don't understand statistics and science or, at the very least, choose not to understand in order to reinforce their prejudices.

About fifty thousand Canadians suffer cardiac arrest or myocardial infarction (heart attacks) each year. Almost 40 percent of them are fatal, meaning twenty thousand deaths. And those are just a fraction of the more than fifty-five thousand deaths from cardiovascular disease in Canada each year. On average, two marathoners a year die during races. Yet they garner more media attention than the thousands of other deaths. Put it down to the man-bites-dog syndrome: the media have a penchant for the unusual, particularly when it occurs in a public venue. And nobody is counting or cataloguing the La-Z-Boy deaths—the thousands of people who die while watching TV or another sedentary activity. But the science is unequivocal: the sedentary—the 50 percent-plus of Canadians who barely move each day—are at greatest risk.

Being active—including running—dramatically decreases your risk of death, particularly from heart disease (which has been edged out by cancer as the country's number-one killer). People who are fit have 50 percent fewer heart attacks than those who are sedentary. They also have a lower risk of stroke, diabetes, cancer and dementia. Being fit does not require feats of super-athleticism. It means upping your heart rate—maybe even working up a sweat—for thirty to sixty minutes a day. That's the equivalent of running (or jogging slowly) about five kilometres for most people.

You don't have to run a marathon to be fit. And you don't have to be Kenyan-marathoner-thin to run either. More than 61 percent of Canadians are overweight or obese, and spectators at any big-city race know marathoners are among those ranks. But running—and, more important, training for a marathon—can make you fitter. To a large extent, it can even offset the risks of being overweight. The research shows that more activity is better for your health. Those whose activity levels surpass the minimum recommended norms tend to have a healthier body weight, lower blood pressure and better cholesterol readings and, overall, they tend to eat better. (Never mind that many marathoners have a voracious appetite and a sweet tooth to boot.) Yes, runners get injured, but their bones are actually stronger and their injuries pale in comparison with those suffered by the obese and the frail.

There are intangibles as well. Marathon and half-marathon participation has exploded in recent years because running is the social activity of choice for many. It is no coincidence that the new runners are predominantly in their thirties and forties—when the fat starts to accumulate around the middle and the prospect of hanging out in bars to make friends becomes depressing. Running is not about vanity; it is about being part of a community and being good to oneself. Public policy should encourage Canadians to be active. Building running trails, bike paths and sidewalks is one of the best investments in health promotion we can make. So, too, is promoting marathons, bike tours, inline-skating races and whatnot—even if it does inconvenience car drivers occasionally.

It would be a shame if the legions of Canadians who are joining running groups at the YMCA, the Running Room and countless other spots were misled into thinking that running is deadly. And it would be downright tragic to slap them with dissuasive measures such as pre-race screening or medical tests. Doing so would be expensive, intrusive and ineffective. The reality is that about 95 percent of those who die during marathons have underlying heart problems—either genetic or lifestyle-related. A surprisingly high number of people have heart abnormalities, but most are benign. Detection does not lessen the risk of death, except in some specific instances. As for the lifestyle-related problems—high blood pressure and high cholesterol—these conditions are commonplace and runners are no exception. That's why a lot of them run in the first place. But predicting the risk of a heart attack during a specific activity is almost impossible.

Paradoxically, if you're going to have a heart attack, a marathon is one of the best places to have one because paramedics and defibrillators are nearby. About 75 percent of people who experience heart stoppage at a race survive; in everyday life, the survival rate for out-of-hospital cardiac arrest is less than 15 percent. (The survival rate from out-of-hospital heart attack, where arteries are blocked but blood flow doesn't stop completely, is considerably higher.) Ultimately, runners and non-runners alike owe it to themselves to go beyond the headlines and retain the important data. Donald Redelmeier, a professor of medicine at the University of Toronto, examined records from marathons with 3.3 million participants over a thirty-year period. There were twenty-six deaths. That's a death rate of one in 126,000—roughly the same as the death rate in the general population. Stated plainly, people die of heart disease, not running. (And, to repeat, being fit reduces the risk of heart disease substantially.)

It is well known that Jim Fixx, whose seminal work *The Complete Book of Running* is credited with sparking the running craze in the 1970s, died of a heart attack while running. Less well known is that he had an underlying heart condition. Doctors estimate that he would have died a decade earlier had he not been fit. Fixx would no doubt be bemused by the debate about the safety of marathons. But his philosophy still holds true today: "I don't know if running adds years to your life, but it adds life to your years."

Get up and get moving

Sitting is the new smoking. Get used to that expression because you're going to be hearing it a lot. Inactivity has become public enemy number one. The reason sedentary behaviour is so worrisome is well illustrated by a study published in October 2012. The research, led by Dr. Emma Wilmot of the diabetes research group at the University of Leicester in Britain, analyzed eighteen existing studies involving almost 800,000 people. The paper, published in the medical journal *Diabetologia*, compared disease rates between the most active and least active among a broad cross-section of adults.

The researchers found that the least active, essentially those who sit all day, had a:

· 147 percent increased risk of heart attack or stroke;
· 112 percent increase in the risk of developing diabetes;
· 90 percent greater risk of dying from a cardiac event; and a
· 49 percent greater risk of premature mortality.

Those are sobering numbers, especially when you consider that the average Canadian adult spends 50 to 70 percent of their daily lives sitting, and roughly another 30 percent sleeping. Do the math and you quickly realize that between sitting in our cars, sitting at our desks at work, sitting in front of the TV, sitting in front of our games consoles, sitting to eat and sitting in school, we hardly move any more. And there is good evidence that inactivity now kills more people than smoking each year. The lack of activity in our daily lives is taking a real toll on our health, individually and collectively.

In recent years, the focus has been on the staggering increase in the number of people who are overweight and obese. That discussion was refined a bit with an emphasis on belly size and waist-to-hip ratio—recognition of where we put on weight matters. But weight is only part of the story. You can be fat and fit, and you can be thin and unfit. What is highly unlikely is, regardless of your body shape, that you are sedentary and healthy. Activity really matters—to your heart, to your brain, to your bones and to your sexual health. It's important, too, to recognize what activity means. It's about moving. You don't have to run a marathon every day to derive health benefits.

Ideally, you should be moderately active—the equivalent of a brisk walk—thirty to sixty minutes a day, every day. But very few people are meeting that minimal standard. According to Statistics

Canada, only 15 percent of adults and 7 percent of children meet the minimum recommended physical activity guidelines every day. Those are the most active people in modern society, and they're not that active. What is even more important than this planned activity is what researchers call "light ambulation"—moving around at regular intervals instead of remaining on your duff. Exercising like a maniac for an hour a day isn't going to offset twenty-three hours of being sedentary. But breaking up your sitting with activity, even very light activity, can have a significant impact.

Take this example, from Wilmot's paper: prolonged sitting sharply reduces glucose and insulin secretion, key factors in developing diabetes. But these changes can be offset by standing and walking two minutes for every twenty minutes of sitting. This is true even in obese people. What this means, practically speaking, is that even if you watch TV for hours at a time, if you get up and walk during the commercials, you will be doing your heart a big favour. Sure, it's even better if you switch off the TV and take the dog for a walk, but even a little effort matters. Similarly, office workers can offset much of their risk by taking a short walk every half-hour, or by having a standing desk, or even by sitting on an exercise ball. Research shows those workers will also be more productive.

Activity has four main components: domestic physical activity, work-related activity, transportation-related activity and exercise. In the past generation or two, levels of activity in each of these areas have fallen sharply—except exercise. From time immemorial until a few decades ago, almost all physical activity occurred during daily work. Today, the number of people doing manual labour has plummeted, while the number of people in white-collar jobs has soared. Manual tasks in the home have also largely disappeared. We vacuum instead of sweep, we have dishwashers instead of washing dishes by hand and we have tractors to cut the lawn. And so on. Almost all our transport is now by car. Fewer than 10 percent of people walk or take public transport to work. The same is true of kids—90 percent are transported to school; they don't walk or bike.

A small—but growing—minority of the population does exercise.

They run, they swim, they do CrossFit or spinning or whatever the latest trendy exercise is. But we are not going to exercise our way out of the real health crisis—sedentary behaviour or, more accurately, sitting disease. The solution is simple movement, a little bit at a time, incorporated into our daily lives. In short, we need to reintroduce a dose of inconvenience into our lives. But we need to think of it not as inconvenience but as a few steps to a better life.

Climate change poses a significant threat to public health

Climate change is the greatest global health threat of the twenty-first century. That is the blunt view of Dr. James Orbinski, a founding member of both Médecins Sans Frontières (Doctors Without Borders) and Dignitas International. At the 2016 general council meeting of the Canadian Medical Association, he presented delegates with a grim catalogue of the health impacts of climate change, including a rise in infectious disease, drought and rising water levels that cause mass displacement, and even violent conflict. But worst of all, he said, "Climate change is a threat that magnifies other threats." Orbinski urged physicians to use their privileged position in society to take a leading role in the public-policy debate because every one of their patients will be affected in some way. "Responding to climate change is not just a scientific or technological issue," he said. "It's time for the CMA to step up and step out, to be genuinely courageous on climate change."

While a small core of self-interested deniers gets a lot of attention, the impacts of climate change are real and undeniable. Countering it will not be easy, but the starting point has to be acknowledging scientific evidence. Since the Industrial Revolution, human activities—particularly the burning of fossil fuels—have released large quantities of carbon dioxide and other greenhouse gases, and that has trapped additional heat in the lower atmosphere and affected the global climate. This phenomenon accelerated in recent decades as the use of fossil fuels soared with increased industrial output, production of motor vehicles and the popularity of air travel. In the last 130 years, the world has warmed by approximately 0.85 degrees Celsius, averaged over land and ocean surfaces, according to the Intergovernmental Panel on Climate Change. While that may not seem like much, the Earth is a fragile and complex ecosystem. As temperatures rise—even a smidgen—glaciers melt, sea levels rise and precipitation patterns change. Climate change used to be called global warming, but it's more complicated than that—extreme weather events of all types are becoming more intense and frequent.

Climate change affects the most fundamental social and environmental determinants of health—clean air, safe drinking water, food security and secure shelter. Globally, the number of reported weather-related natural disasters has more than tripled since the 1960s. Every year, these disasters result in over sixty thousand deaths, mostly in developing countries. When you consider that more than half of the world's population lives within sixty kilometres of the sea, rising sea levels have the potential to be catastrophic. Changing rainfall patterns are increasing the frequency and intensity of drought, sparking famines and compromising access to safe drinking water. In the Darfur region of Sudan, for example, tensions between farmers and herders over disappearing pasture land and evaporating water holes have degenerated into violent clashes and civil war. Orbinski described Darfur as the "world's first climate-change war" and warned that there could be many more to come.

The world is in the midst of an unprecedented refugee crisis—with sixty million people worldwide displaced—and increasingly those mass movements are driven by drought and climate change. Climatic conditions strongly affect water-borne diseases and diseases transmitted through insects, snails or other cold-blooded animals. Climate change is likely to lengthen the reach and breadth of many vector-borne diseases like malaria and dengue, and give rise to new outbreaks, like Zika.

While developing countries will be hardest hit by climate change, developed countries like Canada will feel the impact too. Extreme temperatures, hot and cold, raise the levels of ozone and pollutants in the air and contribute directly to deaths from cardiovascular and respiratory disease, particularly among elderly people. In the heat wave of summer 2003 in Europe, for example, more than seventy thousand "excess deaths" were recorded—meaning more deaths than would normally have been expected to occur in that period. Climate change is more extreme at the poles, and Canada, being a northern country, is seeing temperatures rise at twice the global average. That is having dramatic impacts, especially in the Far North and the country's coastal regions. "There are real questions about the viability of Vancouver as a city due to rising sea levels in coming decades," Orbinski said.

Measuring the health effects from climate change is very approximate; these sorts of predictions are not easy. Nevertheless, it's worth noting that the World Health Organization estimates that, assuming continued economic growth and continued progress in preventing infectious and chronic diseases, climate change will cause 250,000 additional deaths annually between 2030 and 2050. That number includes 38,000 due to heat exposure in elderly people, 48,000 due to diarrhea, 60,000 due to malaria, and 95,000 due to child malnutrition.

In addition to health impacts, there will be economic costs to climate change, and those are potentially staggering. While the cost of reducing emissions is high, the price tag for doing nothing is even higher—an estimated US$1.9 trillion annually by 2100. The Natural Resources Defense Council, a non-profit environmental group, estimates that climate change could take a bite out of economies worth almost 4 percent of gross domestic product. In Canada, that's equivalent to the entire transportation sector.

Given those grim statistics, it's easy to be pessimistic—nihilistic even. But adaptation and mitigation is possible—and essential—from reducing greenhouse gas emissions through to shifting urban areas away from coastlines. The longer we wait, the more painful, expensive and deadly the consequences will be.

CHAPTER 14

Social Determinants

Tips for better living—for
individuals, and society

Every day in the media, you can read reports on the latest health research findings. Many of these articles, implicitly or explicitly, offer advice on how to improve your health: walk more to prevent dementia, eat more tomatoes to stave off prostate cancer, get regular mammograms to reduce the risk of breast cancer and so on. Based on this kind of research, it's easy enough to put together a Letterman-like Top 10 List for Better Living. It would read something like this:

1) Don't smoke.
2) Eat a balanced diet.
3) Be physically active.
4) Limit your stress.
5) If you drink alcohol, do so in moderation.
6) Cover up in the sun.
7) Practice safer sex.
8) Get a regular checkup, including screening for common diseases.
9) Drive carefully: wear a seatbelt and respect speed limits.
10) Learn first aid and CPR.

All these measures relate to lifestyle. But we have long known that there are more important factors in determining your health, including genetics and the environment in which you live. The environment, which academics like to call the socio-economic determinants of health, entered the mainstream in 1974, when then–minister of health and welfare Marc Lalonde issued his landmark report, *New Perspectives on the Health of Canadians*. Forty years on, that perspective is more important than ever, but still largely overlooked. In fact, the factors that have the greatest impact on whether we develop life-threatening diseases are out of our control as individuals.

Income is a far better predictor of heart disease than commitment to regular exercise. The neighbourhood you live in influences your cancer risk more than your diet. The job you work at will give you a much better idea of your Alzheimer's risk than the amount of fish oil you consume. And your level of education will determine your longevity more accurately than screening tests. In other words, general living conditions contribute more to long-term health status and mortality rates than lifestyle practices. Factors like education, income, employment, housing and the environment influence your health as much, if not more, than medical treatment (or more accurately, sickness care).

This has led academics to come up with alternative tips for healthy living. This Top 10 list is from Joan Wharf Higgins, a professor of physical education at the University of Victoria:

1) Don't be poor.
2) Pick your parents well.
3) Graduate from high school or, better yet, university.
4) Don't work at a stressful, low-paid job. Find a job where you have decision-making power and control.
5) Learn to control stress levels.
6) Be able to afford a foreign holiday and sunbathe (with SPF 30).
7) Don't be unemployed.
8) Leave in a community where you have a sense of belonging.
9) Don't live in a ghetto, near a major road or near a polluting factory.
10) Learn to make friends and keep them.

These goals are considerably more difficult to achieve than the usual Top 10. As a result, many find this kind of talk demoralizing because they feel powerless in the face of health threats. But knowing more about the underlying factors influencing our health does not discredit healthy living or absolve people of personal responsibility. Rather, we should be empowered knowing that the social, economic and political choices we make can influence our health, and the health of the population.

If we want a healthy society, we need more than a health-care system that delivers state-of-the-art sickness care. We need an environment and a culture that supports healthy living. The paradox today is that those who could benefit most from lifestyle changes are the least likely to make them. To make healthy choices, you need a decent income, proper housing, adequate nutrition, a good education, a safe neighbourhood, a sense of belonging and a modicum of control over your life.

The countries with the best health outcomes and the highest life expectancy have the smallest income gap between rich and poor. And big gaps in our knowledge of these influences, and our failure to mitigate them as best we can, is equally bad for our health. We are fooling ourselves if we think the promotion of healthy lifestyles will have an impact unless an equal or greater dedication is made to creating a society in which we each have the opportunity to make healthy choices.

Health's a black-and-white issue: Colour-blindness is killing minorities

While February is Black History Month, any month is a good time to reflect on the inequalities that persist in society. In particular, we need to ponder the question, what impact does inequality have on the health of individuals and on the health of the society they live in?

Research published in the February 2005 edition of the *American Journal of Public Health* is a good starting point. Dr. Steven Woolf, director of research in the department of family medicine at Virginia Commonwealth University in Richmond, Virginia, calculated that between 1991 and 2000, a staggering 886,000 deaths could have been prevented had African-Americans received the same care as whites. But Woolf and his team didn't stop there. They calculated that technological improvements in medicine—better drugs, new medical devices, improved surgical procedures—averted 176,633 deaths in the general population during that same period.

What this means, practically speaking, is that five times as many lives could be saved by correcting the disparities in care between blacks and whites than in developing fancy new treatments. "The prudence of investing billions in the development of new drugs and technologies, while investing only a fraction of that amount in the correction of disparities, deserves reconsideration. It is an imbalance that may claim more lives than it saves," Woolf said.

His study found that, in the United States, the cancer rate for African-Americans was 25 percent higher than for whites; blacks were twice as likely to die of diabetes; the infant mortality rate among blacks was more than twice as high as among whites; adult African-Americans were half as likely as whites to be immunized against diseases such as influenza; blacks were eleven times more likely than whites to die of HIV-AIDS and nine times as likely to be victims of murder; the age-adjusted mortality rates were about 30 percent higher across the board for blacks than whites. These troubling statistics prompted a lot more research and some action but, a decade later, the situation was only marginally better.

A 2014 report from the Robert Wood Johnson Foundation found that 40 percent of African-Americans receive worse health care than whites, they have more illness and shorter lives, and these disparities cost the economy more than US$60 billion. The US Department of Health and Human Services produced a similarly sobering report in 2015 on racial and ethnic health disparities, though it featured some glimmers of good news. The black–white mortality gap reached its lowest in history—with African-Americans living 3.4 years less on average than whites. One of the main reasons was that the homicide rate for black men had plummeted, from 78 per 100,000 to 31 per 100,000; another was that the number of white people dying from opioid-related deaths soared.

Blacks do not have worse health outcomes because of the darker pigmentation of their skin. Generally speaking, they have poorer health outcomes because they have lower incomes, higher rates of unemployment, disproportionate rates of imprisonment and substandard housing, and because they are far more likely to live in neighbourhoods that are polluted, that have poor educational facilities and even worse health facilities. In the United States, access to health care is, of course, also an issue of dollars and cents. About twenty-nine million Americans do not have access to health care because they cannot afford it—and a disproportionate number of them are black. But there was progress here too: about twenty million people who were uninsured were able to purchase coverage because of the Affordable Care Act (known commonly as Obamacare), including 2.3 million African-Americans.

But Canadians should not fool themselves into thinking that because we have a universal health system, access to care is equal. There is ample evidence that it is not. Even though medically necessary care itself is "free," getting timely treatment for yourself and family members requires a certain level of education, the ability to get time off work, transportation and so on. Health facilities are better in wealthier neighbourhoods, and all sorts of treatments, such as prescription drugs, require out-of-pocket spending.

So there is no reason to believe that the health outcomes of blacks in Canada are dramatically different from those in the United States. (Though we don't know for sure because of an absence of research. In Canada, we have been squeamish about exploring racial and cultural differences in health outcomes. While this colour-blindness is laudable, it is probably interfering with the need to address racial disparities in health care.) The 2005 US research, by implication, tells us that the benefits of technological advances are going disproportionately to the wealthy, to whites. When billions are invested in new technologies, they are not trickling down to all levels of society quickly enough. When there are shortages of health dollars—and there always will be—those with the least political clout, notably visible minorities and the poor, will suffer. This translates into insufficient resources for communities that most need the extra help, and unequal use of proven interventions. But medical care is only a small part of what makes people and communities healthy. The US research serves as a poignant reminder that the best way to improve the overall health of a population is to tackle the underlying socio-economic determinants of health—income, job security, housing, the environment and a sense of belonging.

For too many racial and ethnic minorities, good health remains elusive. It remains so because we have not done enough to target programs at specific groups such as African-Canadians and African-Americans, including everything from social welfare to health-promotion campaigns. Doing so can be difficult, and it can make us uncomfortable. But it is necessary to improve the health outcomes of blacks and other minorities in our multicultural society. As civil rights leader Martin Luther King said, "Our lives begin to end the day we become silent about things that matter." In Black History Month and all year round, we need to be reminded that our silence on the issue of the health of African-Canadians and -Americans is proving deadly.

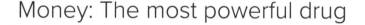

Money: The most powerful drug

Life expectancy in Canada rivals that of almost any country in the world. A girl born in Canada today can expect to live, on average, to 83.6 and a boy to a more modest 79.4, according to Statistics Canada (2012). But life expectancy is a crude measure that tells a superficial story, so there have been many attempts to drill down into the data.

There are, for example, wide regional variations. In Canada, there is a west-to-east-to-north health gradient: those who are healthiest and live longest are on the Pacific Coast, and the numbers get gradually worse as you move across the nation to the Atlantic region. Then, when you look to the north, the numbers take a precipitous drop. In the territories, life expectancy is similar to that in low- and middle-income countries.

Just as there are regional variations, there are differences across the lifespan. Those who die early tend to skew data on average life expectancy. This has given rise to the popular measure of life expectancy at sixty-five. On her sixty-fifth birthday, a Canadian woman can expect to live twenty-two more years on average, and a man almost nineteen (2012).

Increasingly, those years are lived in good health. But a significant number of seniors have chronic health conditions. According to Statistics Canada, Canadians, on average, start to experience "activity limitations" at age sixty-nine, and "severe activity limitations" at age seventy-seven. There is even a measure, disability-free life expectancy (DFLE), that allows us to look beyond mortality to the preceding morbidity. In 2007, the most recent year for which data are available, a fifty-year-old woman could expect to live 34.5 more years, 26.5 of those disability-free. That means she could expect to live 8 years with severe disability. A fifty-year-old man, by comparison, could expect to live 30.7 more years, 26.8 of them disability-free. That translates to 3.9 years, on average, with a severe disability.

In other words, the increases in life expectancy we've seen in recent decades don't tend to be healthy years. Most people can expect to live the last four to eight years of their lives needing significant help with the activities of daily living—meaning institutional living or considerable amounts of home care.

But that is only the tip of the iceberg. Health tends to decline gradually, not suddenly. So Statistics Canada has developed another measure, health-adjusted life-expectancy (HALE) that looks beyond longevity to quality of life. Essentially, it's a scoring system that looks at factors such as pain and mobility and is used to weight the years lived in good health higher than years lived in poor health.

A study published in the March 2013 edition of *Health Reports* shows that older Canadians can expect to live the last decade or so of their lives with serious illness, and a couple of more decades if they have a significant chronic illness like diabetes. For example, a woman with a life expectancy of 83.6 years has a disability-free life expectancy of 72.1 years, and of 58.1 years if she suffers from diabetes and hypertension. For a man with a life expectancy of 78.9, the disability-free number is 69.6, and just 56 when saddled with hypertension and diabetes.

It is well established that many variables contribute to poor health. In addition to genetics (which plays a relatively small role), socio-economic status and, to a lesser extent, lifestyle choices have a tremendous impact. Those socio-economic determinants include education, housing, physical environment and, above all, income. Put bluntly, poverty makes people unhealthy and poverty kills.

While this may seem self-evident, a group of researchers at Statistics Canada has managed to calculate the impact of poverty (or, as they say, "income disparities") on life expectancy. Only 51.2 percent of Canadian men in the lowest income group (the bottom 10 percent) can expect to live to age seventy-five. By comparison, 74.6 percent of high-income earners (the top 10 percent) can expect to see seventy-five. That is a startling 23.4-point difference—not good odds. For women, the comparative figures are 69.4 percent of poor women living to seventy-five, compared with 84.4 percent of wealthy women—a smaller but still significant 15-point gap. Put another way, at age twenty-five a poor man can expect to live an additional 48.6 years. A wealthy man can expect an additional 56 years—a 7.4-year gap. A poor twenty-five-year-old woman can be expected to live 56.5 more years, compared with 61 years for a wealthy woman of the same age. That gap is 4.5 years.

Those are the raw numbers based on conventional life expectancy. When Statistics Canada applied the HALE measure, it found that those gaps between poor and rich were even more considerable. Being wealthy translated into 11.4 more years of healthy living for men and 9.7 for women. When they crunched the numbers further, the statisticians found that even if you compare the health-adjusted life expectancy of the highest-income earners with those of the average person, the difference was still 5.9 years for men and 4.2 years for women. To put those numbers in context, consider that cancer, the number-one killer in Canada, reduces health-adjusted life expectancy by just 2.8 years for men and 2.5 years for women.

There are a lot of numbers to digest here, but the bottom line is this: people's income (or lack thereof) has about twice the impact on their health as cancer does. These data are as humbling as they are informative. They are also greatly underused. They should be guiding how we plan for the provision of health and social services—from setting social assistance rates at a level that allows people to live healthily through to planning for more home care and long-term care for seniors.

The numbers should also lead us to ask the question, why is tackling poverty not a health priority? Patching and mending is all well and good, and our sickness-care system does a good job of it. But the data tell us that the best tool we have in our health-care armamentarium is income redistribution. The most powerful drug we have—money—is pretty plentiful in Canada. But it is not being prescribed to everyone who would benefit.

Life expectancy is a crude measurement, just as medicine is a crude method of making people healthier. What determines how long we live, and how well we live, is not fancy technologies; it is whether we have a roof over our heads, sufficient food and a sense of contribution and belonging.

If there is a message to retain from this collection of essays, a bit of wisdom that emerges from my more than three decades of health journalism, it is that, in life and in death, it is the little things that matter. Good health and a good health system often don't require grand gestures, but rather a relentless focus on the basics. We can't live forever, but, with increased individual awareness and improved government policies, we can try to live the lives we have well, and meaningfully.

Acknowledgements

First and foremost, I must thank *The Globe and Mail* for allowing me to collect and collate this selection of columns in book form. Without the permission and support of editor-in-chief David Walmsley and publisher Phillip Crawley this book would not have been possible. I hope the end product reflects well on the paper.

As I pored through the archives looking for columns to include, I was reminded how privileged I am to work for Canada's national newspaper. Not only do I have a column in the paper and online—some of the most precious real estate in journalism anywhere in the world—but I get to work with fabulous editors, each and every day.

Over my more than thirty years at *The Globe*, I have worked with many editors, but one stands out. Paul Taylor, the paper's long-time health editor, always made my copy better and (almost) always caught my mistakes before they were revealed to the world. His invisible fingerprints are all over this book.

The columns collected here were written over a period of about fifteen years. The data has changed, governments have fallen and some of the language we use has evolved, so many updates were required. I was lucky to have the keen eye and sharp pen of editor Arlene Prunkl to guide me through the process.

I write about a vast range of health topics, but I am an expert in none. I depend on the kindness and generosity of countless researchers, policy-makers and health professionals to help me understand and explain complex issues. They make me sound a lot smarter than I am.

As a columnist—someone who expresses opinions—I invariably and routinely anger and irritate people. But, with very few exceptions, my readers have always been kind and polite. There are few things more quintessentially Canadian than respectful, apologetic disagreement.

Thank you for reading for the past thirty years. Hopefully, in the years to come, there will be many more columns to read and, I'm sorry to say, to sometimes disagree with.

Index

insurance, health (*cont.*)

    premiums, 21–22, 23

    private, 20, 37, 38

    public, 38

    See also medicare; Obamacare

journalism and health, 7–13, 83, 117,
    154, 257, 267

    reporting on physician-assisted
      death, 121, 127

    reporting on suicide, 56–58,
      58–60, 61, 68–70

    reporting on infectious diseases,
      8–9, 234, 239–41

Kelley, Frances, 180

Kirby, Michael, 54, 66–68

Lancet, the, 91, 140, 156, 158–59

lead poisoning, 134–36

leukemia, 200, 215, 249

Liberal Party of Canada, 73

    See also Government of Canada

lifestyle, 245–64, 267–69

    See also climate change; diet;
      exercise; smoking; weight

literacy, 137–39

    Reach Out and Read, 137

    See also education

lung disease, 239, 264

    Canadian Lung Association,
      237, 253

    chronic obstructive pulmonary
      disease (COPD), 249, 252–53

    Montreal Chest Institute, 32

Manitoba, 194

marijuana. *See* cannabis

maternity, 142–44

    See also reproductive health

McGill University, 45, 232

media, the. *See* journalism and health

medical school, 61–63

medicare, 17–24, 25, 26–28, 107–9,
    133, 152, 238

    coverage, 66, 247 (*see also* drugs,
      prescription: coverage of)

    delivery of, 18–19, 22, 35, 38,
      39–40 (*see also* patient-
      centred care)

    funding of, 19–20, 36–38, 39,
      42, 224

    privatization of, 22, 36–37

    rural–urban split in, 26–28

    services of, 23, 38, 66, 72, 152

    See also insurance, health

mental health, 49–78, 101, 111, 123,
    126, 127

    At Home/Chez Soi research
      project, 67

    Bill C-300, 67

    Centre for Addiction and
      Mental Health, 87–88

    community treatment orders
      (CTOs), 63–65

    Consent and Capacity Board, 64

    eating disorders, *see* eating
      disorders

    Empowerment Council Systemic
      Advocates in Addictions
      and Mental Health, 63